HEALTHY MEAL PREP COOKBOOK 2024

Unlock the Secrets to Easy, Balanced Eating Every Day

By

Hector Wiggins

Table of Contents

INTRODUCTION

In the bustling heart of a modern kitchen, where the aroma of fresh herbs dances amidst the clatter of pots and pans, lies the gateway to a culinary revolution. Welcome to the "Healthy Meal Prep Cookbook 2024," a vibrant tapestry of flavors, nourishment, and the artistry of meal preparation.

Picture this: a world where hectic schedules no longer dictate the quality of your meals, where the rush of daily life is seamlessly integrated with the serenity of mindful eating. This cookbook isn't just about recipes; it's a journey—a journey that begins with a simple notion: the power of preparation.

In these pages, you'll embark on a voyage to reclaim control over your diet and well-being. Here, meal prep isn't merely a chore—it's a form of self-care, a mindful act of nurturing your body and soul.
It's about savoring the process as much as relishing the final dish.

Join us as we delve into the art of crafting nutritious meals ahead of time, transforming your kitchen into a sanctuary of health and vitality. From the crisp pages of this cookbook emerge recipes that tantalize the taste buds while honoring your body's need for wholesome nourishment.

But our journey doesn't stop at the kitchen counter. With each recipe, we'll explore the stories behind the ingredients, the cultural influences that shape our culinary landscape, and the science that underpins the magic of healthy eating.

As you flip through these pages, envision the possibilities: vibrant salads that sing with freshness, hearty stews that warm the soul, and decadent desserts that indulge without guilt. Here, healthy eating isn't a sacrifice—it's a celebration of life, a symphony of flavors that awaken the senses and nourish the body from within.

So, my dear reader, let this cookbook serve as your road map—a source of motivation and direction on your quest for wellbeing—regardless of your level of experience in the kitchen. Let's set out on a gastronomic adventure where each dish is a work of art and each mouthful serves as a celebration of the joys of leading a healthy lifestyle. This is the "Healthy Meal Prep Cookbook 2024"—a place where delicious cuisine and optimal health combine to provide a delightful and nourishing experience.

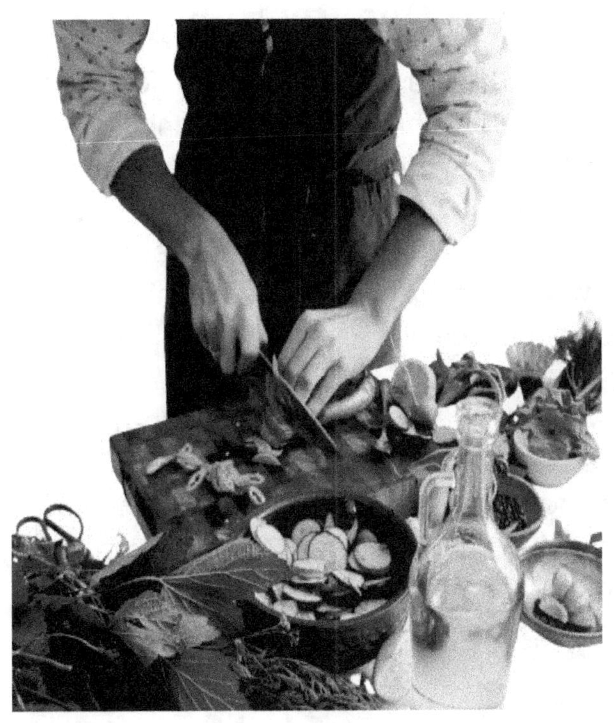

Welcome to Healthy Eating

In the fast-paced rhythm of modern life, finding the balance between nourishment and convenience can often feel like a daunting task. But fear not, for you've just stepped into the world of Healthy Meal Prep—a sanctuary where wholesome eating and efficiency harmoniously coexist.

Here, we believe that preparation is the cornerstone of a vibrant, nourished life. By dedicating a bit of time and effort upfront, you can unlock a treasure trove of benefits: from saving time and money to effortlessly maintaining a nutritious diet throughout the week.

Welcome to a realm where the kitchen becomes your playground, and meal prep transforms from a chore into a joyful ritual. Embrace the rhythm of chopping vegetables, the sizzle of sautéing proteins, and the aroma of spices mingling in perfect harmony.

In these pages, you'll discover a treasure trove of recipes designed to streamline your cooking process without compromising on flavor or nutrition. From vibrant salads to hearty stews, from wholesome breakfasts to satisfying snacks, each recipe is crafted with care to nourish your body and delight your taste buds.

But Healthy Meal Prep is more than just recipes—it's a lifestyle. It's about reclaiming control over your diet, empowering yourself to make healthier choices, and savoring the satisfaction of nourishing your body from within.

So, whether you're a busy professional, a dedicated parent, or simply someone who values their health and time, welcome to Healthy Meal Prep. Together, let's embark on a journey to wellness—one deliciously prepared meal at a time.

Benefits of Meal Prep

Meal prep offers a multitude of benefits, making it a popular strategy for individuals looking to streamline their cooking routine and maintain a healthier lifestyle. Here are some of the key benefits of meal prep:

Time Savings: By preparing meals in advance, you can significantly reduce the amount of time spent cooking during busy weekdays. With pre-prepared meals on hand, you can simply reheat and enjoy, saving precious time that can be allocated to other priorities.

Consistency: Meal prep promotes consistency in your diet by ensuring that you have nutritious meals readily available throughout the week. This consistency can help you stay on track with your health and nutrition goals, whether you're trying to lose weight, build muscle, or simply eat more balanced meals.

Portion Control: Portion sizes can be a challenge to manage, especially when eating out or preparing meals on the fly. With meal prep, you have control over portion sizes, allowing you to better manage your calorie intake and maintain a healthy weight.

Cost Savings: Eating out or ordering takeout regularly can quickly add up, both in terms of cost and calories. Meal prep allows you to buy ingredients in bulk, cook in larger quantities, and portion out meals ahead of time, ultimately saving you money and reducing food waste.

Healthier Choices: When you have pre-prepared meals on hand, you're less likely to succumb to unhealthy convenience foods or impulsive eating decisions. Meal prep empowers you to make healthier choices by ensuring that nutritious options are readily available and easily accessible.

Reduced Stress: The daily hustle and bustle of life can be stressful enough without the added pressure of figuring out what to eat for each meal. Meal prep takes the guesswork out of mealtime, reducing stress and promoting a sense of calm and control in your daily routine.

Customization: With meal prep, you have the flexibility to customize your meals according to your dietary preferences, restrictions, and nutritional needs. Whether you follow a specific diet like keto, vegetarian, or gluten-free, or simply prefer certain flavors and ingredients, meal prep allows you to tailor your meals to suit your individual tastes.

Improved Food Quality: When you prepare your meals at home, you have full control over the quality of ingredients you use. You can choose fresh, whole foods, and prioritize organic or locally sourced ingredients, resulting in meals that are not only nutritious but also free from additives, preservatives, and other unhealthy additives commonly found in processed foods.

Enhanced Energy Levels: Consistently fueling your body with balanced, nutritious meals through meal prep can lead to sustained energy levels throughout the day. By avoiding energy crashes associated with high-sugar or high-fat meals, you'll experience improved focus, productivity, and overall well-being.

Encourages Mindful Eating: Meal prep encourages mindful eating by promoting a deeper connection with your food. When you take the time to plan, prepare, and portion out your meals in advance, you become more aware of what you're consuming and can savor each bite mindfully. This can lead to a greater appreciation for food, reduced overeating, and a more positive relationship with eating and nourishment.

How to Use This Cookbook

Using the "Healthy Meal Prep Cookbook" is a straightforward and rewarding process, designed to empower you to take control of your nutrition and simplify your cooking routine. Here's a guide on how to make the most of this cookbook:

Read the Introduction: Start by reading the introduction section of the cookbook. This will provide you with valuable insights into the philosophy behind healthy meal prep, as well as tips and techniques to help you get started.

Familiarize Yourself with the Layout: Take a moment to familiarize yourself with the layout of the cookbook. You'll typically find chapters dedicated to different meal categories, such as breakfast, lunch, dinner, snacks, and desserts. Each chapter may also include special dietary options or tips for success.

Choose Your Recipes: Browse through the recipes and select the ones that appeal to you. Pay attention to any dietary preferences or restrictions you may have, and choose recipes that align with your needs.

Create a Meal Plan: Once you've selected your recipes, create a meal plan for the week. Consider factors such as your schedule, the number of servings you'll need, and any ingredients you already have on hand. Planning ahead will help streamline your cooking process and ensure you have everything you need.

Make a Shopping List: Based on your meal plan, create a shopping list of ingredients you'll need to purchase. This will help you stay organized and ensure you have everything you need when it's time to cook.

Prep Ingredients in Advance: Before you start cooking, take some time to prep your ingredients. This may include chopping vegetables, marinating proteins, or cooking grains. By prepping ingredients in advance, you'll save time during the cooking process and make meal prep more efficient.

Follow the Recipes: When it's time to cook, follow the recipes in the cookbook step by step. Pay attention to measurements, cooking times, and any special instructions provided. Feel free to customize the recipes to suit your taste preferences or dietary needs.

Meal Preparation and Storage: After your meals are prepared, divide them into little portions and keep them chilled or frozen. To keep yourself organized, put the name of the dish and the preparation date on the label of each container.

Enjoy Your Meals: Throughout the week, simply reheat and enjoy your pre-prepared meals. Sit back, relax, and savor the delicious flavors and nourishing ingredients that you've prepared with care.

By following these steps, you'll be able to seamlessly integrate the recipes from the "Healthy Meal Prep Cookbook" into your daily routine, making healthy eating easier and more enjoyable than ever before.

CHAPTER ONE

Getting Started with Meal Prep

Getting started with meal prep is an empowering journey towards efficiency, health, and culinary creativity. Whether you're a seasoned meal prepper or just beginning to explore this method of cooking, understanding the basics is essential to your success. Here's a comprehensive guide to help you get started with meal prep:

Understand Meal Prep Basics: Meal prep involves preparing meals or meal components in advance, typically for several days or the entire week. This can include chopping vegetables, cooking grains or proteins, and assembling dishes to be stored and reheated later. The key is to streamline the cooking process and make healthy eating more convenient.

Gather Essential Tools and Equipment:
Before diving into meal prep, make sure you have the necessary tools and equipment on hand. This may include food storage containers, meal prep trays or pans, sharp knives, cutting boards, and kitchen utensils. Investing in quality tools will make the meal prep process smoother and more efficient.

Plan Your Meals: Start by planning your meals for the week ahead. Consider your schedule, dietary preferences, and nutritional goals when choosing recipes. Aim for a balance of proteins, carbohydrates, and healthy fats, and incorporate plenty of fruits and vegetables for added vitamins and minerals.

Make a Grocery List: Once you've planned your meals, create a grocery list of ingredients you'll need to purchase. Organize your list by category (e.g., produce, proteins, pantry staples) to make shopping easier and more efficient. Stick to your list to avoid impulse purchases and ensure you have everything you need for the week.

Set Aside Time for Prep: Dedicate a block of time each week to meal prep. This could be a few hours on the weekend or a weeknight evening when you have some free time. Choose a time when you're not rushed and can fully focus on cooking and preparing meals.

Prep Ingredients in Advance: Before you start cooking, prep your ingredients by washing, chopping, and portioning them as needed. This will make the cooking process smoother and save time during meal prep. Consider batch cooking staple ingredients like grains, proteins, and sauces to use in multiple meals throughout the week.

Cook and Assemble Meals: Once your ingredients are prepped, start cooking your meals according to your recipes. Cook in bulk to save time and energy, and consider using sheet pans or one-pot recipes to minimize cleanup. Assemble your meals in individual containers, portioning them out according to your needs.

Store and Reheat Meals: Once your meals are cooked and assembled, store them in the refrigerator or freezer until you're ready to eat. Label each container with the name of the dish and the date it was prepared for easy identification. When you're ready to eat, simply reheat your meals in the microwave or oven and enjoy!

Understanding Meal Prep Basics

Meal prep is the practice of preparing meals in advance, typically for the week ahead. It involves planning, cooking, and storing meals to make eating healthier, more convenient, and cost-effective. Here are some key basics to understand about meal prep:

Planning: Start by deciding what meals you want to prepare for the upcoming week. Consider your dietary preferences, nutritional goals, and any special dietary needs.

Recipes: Choose simple and versatile recipes that can be easily scaled up or down. Look for meals that use similar ingredients to minimize waste and save time.

Grocery Shopping: Make a list of ingredients based on your chosen recipes and stick to it when grocery shopping. This helps to avoid impulse purchases and ensures you have everything you need for meal prep.

Preparation: Schedule a weekly period for preparing meals. This could be a shorter session during the week or a few hours on the weekend. To expedite cooking, wash, cut, and divide out ingredients.

Cooking: Cook large batches of food to portion out into individual meals. Use cooking methods like baking, grilling, or sautéing to prepare proteins, vegetables, and grains.

Storage: Invest in quality storage containers that are microwave and dishwasher safe. Portion out meals into containers and label them with the date and contents for easy identification.

Variety: Keep meals interesting by rotating recipes and incorporating a variety of flavors, textures, and cuisines. This prevents boredom and ensures you're getting a well-balanced diet.

Safety: Practice proper food safety techniques, such as washing hands, cleaning surfaces, and storing perishable items in the refrigerator or freezer promptly.

Adaptability: Be flexible with your meal prep routine and adjust as needed based on changes in schedule, dietary preferences, or ingredient availability.

Enjoyment: Meal prep should simplify your life and make eating healthier more enjoyable. Experiment with new recipes, involve family members, and find joy in nourishing your body with wholesome meals.

Essential Tools and Equipment

Cutting Board and Sharp Knives: A sturdy cutting board and sharp knives are essential for chopping vegetables, fruits, and proteins efficiently and safely.

Meal Prep Containers: Invest in high-quality, reusable containers in various sizes to portion out and store your prepared meals. Look for options that are microwave-safe, dishwasher-safe, and leak-proof.

Cookware Set: A versatile cookware set including pots, pans, and baking sheets allows you to cook a variety of dishes using different cooking methods such as boiling, sautéing, and baking.

Food Processor or Blender: These appliances are handy for chopping, pureeing, and blending ingredients for sauces, dips, smoothies, and more.

Slow Cooker or Instant Pot: These kitchen appliances are excellent for hands-off cooking and can be used to prepare large batches of soups, stews, and one-pot meals with minimal effort.

Steamer Basket: A steamer basket is useful for cooking vegetables while retaining their nutrients and vibrant colors. It's a healthier alternative to boiling or sautéing.

Grill or Grill Pan: Grilling adds flavor to meats, seafood, and vegetables without the need for added fats. A grill or grill pan allows you to prepare lean proteins and grilled vegetables for healthy meal options.

Measuring Cups and Spoons: Accurate measurement is crucial for portion control and maintaining nutritional balance. Invest in a set of measuring cups and spoons for precise ingredient measurements.

Scale: A kitchen scale is useful for measuring ingredients by weight, especially for recipes that require precise measurements for baking or portioning out servings.

Storage Bags and Wrap: Stock up on reusable storage bags, aluminum foil, and plastic wrap for storing prepped ingredients and leftovers. These help maintain freshness and prevent food waste.

Salad Spinner: Washing and drying leafy greens is essential for salads and other dishes. A salad spinner makes it easy to rinse and remove excess moisture from greens, ensuring crisp and fresh salads.

Vegetable Peeler and Spiralizer: These tools make it easy to peel and prepare vegetables in different shapes and sizes, adding variety and creativity to your meals.

Planning Your Meals

Achieving your nutritional goals and guaranteeing success in healthy meal prep requires careful meal planning. Here's how to organize your meals efficiently:

Establish Your Objectives: Identify your dietary requirements and objectives, including maintaining a healthy diet or achieving specific goals like weight loss, muscle gain, or increased energy. You'll make decisions about meal planning based on your goals.

Create a Weekly Menu: Start by planning out your meals for the week ahead. Consider breakfast, lunch, dinner, and snacks. Aim for a balance of macronutrients (carbohydrates, proteins, and fats) and include a variety of fruits, vegetables, whole grains, lean proteins, and healthy fats.

Consider Dietary Preferences and Restrictions: Take into account any dietary preferences or restrictions, such as vegetarian, vegan, gluten-free, or dairy-free options. Plan meals that cater to your preferences while still providing the nutrients your body needs.

Choose Recipes: Select recipes that align with your goals, preferences, and dietary needs. Look for recipes that are nutritious, balanced, and easy to prepare. Consider incorporating one-pot meals, sheet pan dinners, or make-ahead options for added convenience.

Check Your Pantry and Fridge: Take inventory of ingredients you already have on hand and incorporate them into your meal plan. This helps reduce food waste and saves money by using up ingredients before they expire.

Make a Grocery List: Based on your planned meals, create a comprehensive grocery list of ingredients you'll need for the week. Organize your list by food categories (produce, dairy, proteins, etc.) to make shopping more efficient.

Shop Smart: Stick to your grocery list to avoid impulse purchases and stay within your budget. Choose fresh, whole foods whenever possible and opt for organic and locally sourced ingredients if available and affordable.

Prep in Advance: Set aside time for meal prep, whether it's a few hours on the weekend or shorter sessions throughout the week. Wash, chop, and portion out ingredients ahead of time to streamline the cooking process during the week.

Be Flexible: Life happens, and plans may change. Be flexible with your meal plan and willing to adapt as needed. Have backup options on hand, such as frozen meals or pantry staples, for busy days or unexpected events.

Track Your Progress: Keep track of your meals and how they make you feel. Monitor your progress towards your goals and adjust your meal plan as necessary based on feedback from your body.

Grocery Shopping Tips

Plan Ahead: Before heading to the grocery store, take the time to plan your meals for the week. This will help you create a detailed shopping list and avoid unnecessary purchases.

Stick to the List: Once you have your shopping list, stick to it! Avoid impulse buys by focusing only on the items you need for your planned meals. This will help you stay within your budget and prevent food waste.

Shop the Perimeter: The perimeter of the grocery store typically contains fresh produce, lean proteins, dairy, and whole grains. Focus on filling your cart with these nutritious options, while limiting your time in the aisles filled with processed foods.

Select entire Foods: Whenever feasible, choose entire, minimally processed foods. Fruits, vegetables, whole grains, lean meats, and good fats are a few of these. Steer clear of foods heavy in harmful fats, salt, and added sugars.

Examine the labels: Spend some time reading the nutrition labels on packaged goods that you choose. Seek for goods with minimal preservatives, low added sugar content, and brief ingredient lists. Be mindful of portion sizes and choose meals that are high in protein and fiber.

Buying staples in bulk can result in long-term cost savings. Examples of such bulk purchases include grains, beans, nuts, and seeds. To preserve freshness, just be sure to store them correctly in sealed containers.

Consider Seasonal Produce: Seasonal fruits and vegetables are often fresher, tastier, and more affordable. Incorporate seasonal produce into your meal plan to add variety to your meals and support local farmers.

Compare Prices: Compare prices between brands and package sizes to get the best value for your money. Consider buying store-brand or generic items, which are often cheaper than name brands but still of good quality.

Shop for Sales: Keep an eye out for sales, discounts, and coupons on items you regularly use. Stock up on pantry staples and non-perishable items when they're on sale to save money in the long term.

Don't Shop Hungry: Shopping on an empty stomach can lead to impulse buys and unhealthy food choices. Eat a nutritious snack or meal before heading to the grocery store to help you stick to your shopping list and make healthier decisions.

CHAPTER TWO

Breakfast Recipes

Breakfast is often considered the most important meal of the day, and preparing healthy options in advance can set the tone for a nutritious day ahead. Here are some breakfast recipes suitable for meal prep:

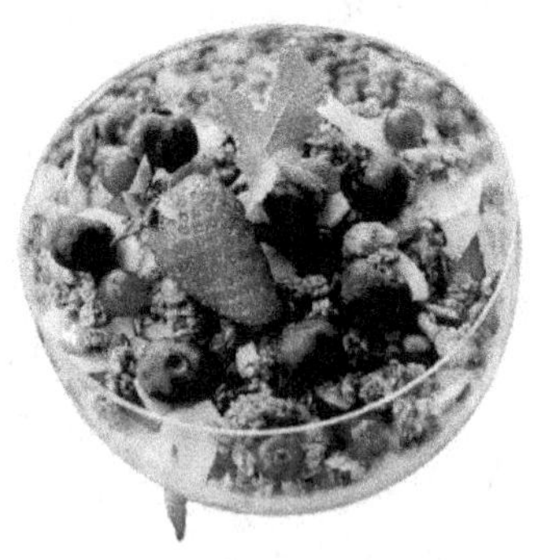

Overnight Oats: In a jar or other container, combine rolled oats with yogurt, chia seeds, your preferred kind of milk (vegan or dairy), and sweetener (such honey or maple syrup). provide spices, nuts, or fruits to provide different flavors. Enjoy it cold or slightly heated in the morning after leaving it in the fridge for the entire night.

Egg Muffins: Beat eggs with cooked proteins (such diced chicken, turkey, or ham) and diced veggies (like bell peppers, spinach, onions, and tomatoes). After filling muffin tins with oil, bake the batter until it sets. These portable egg muffins are perfect for an on-the-go, high-protein breakfast because they reheat quickly.

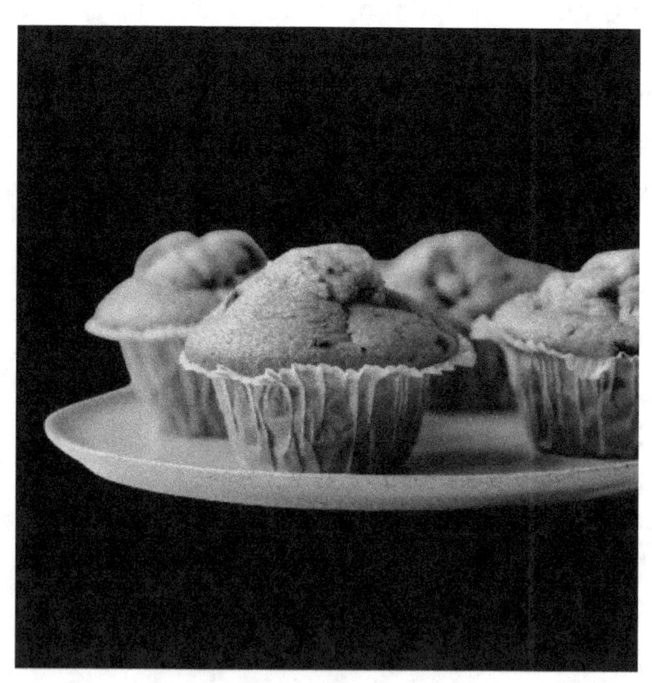

Smoothie Packs: Pre-portion smoothie ingredients into individual freezer bags or containers. Include fruits (such as berries, bananas, and mango), leafy greens (like spinach or kale), protein powder, seeds (such as chia or flaxseed), and liquid (milk, yogurt, or water). In the morning, simply blend the contents with your preferred liquid for a refreshing and nutritious smoothie.

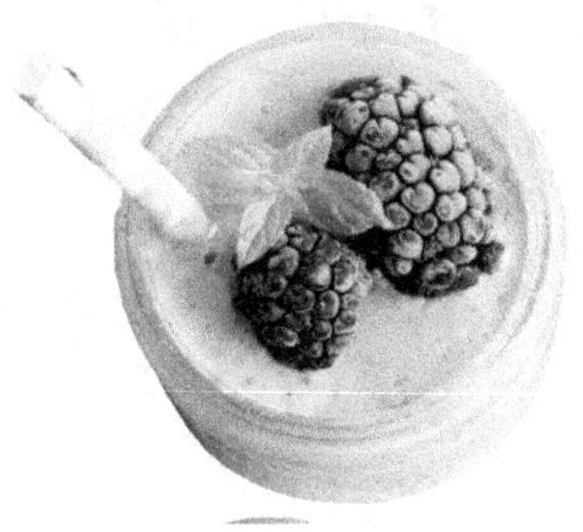

Breakfast Burritos: Fill whole wheat or corn tortillas with scrambled eggs, cooked turkey sausage or bacon, sautéed vegetables, and a sprinkle of cheese. Roll them up and wrap each burrito tightly in foil or plastic wrap. Store them in the refrigerator or freezer, then reheat in the microwave for a satisfying breakfast option.

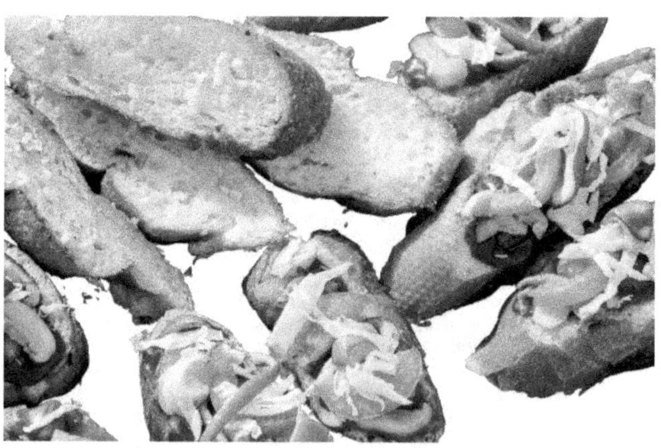

Greek Yogurt Parfaits: Layer Greek yogurt with granola, fresh berries, and a drizzle of honey or maple syrup in individual containers or jars. These creamy and satisfying parfaits can be made ahead and enjoyed cold for a quick and nutritious breakfast.

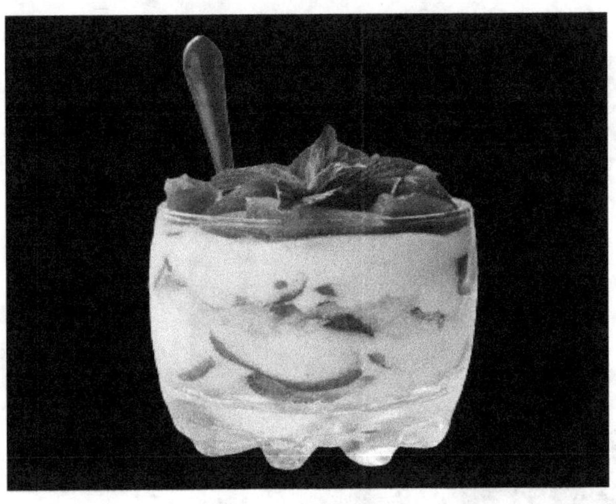

Quinoa Breakfast Bowls: Cook quinoa according to package instructions and portion it into containers. Top each serving with Greek yogurt, sliced bananas or berries, nuts or seeds, and a drizzle of nut butter or honey. Quinoa breakfast bowls are high in protein and fiber, providing long-lasting energy to start your day.

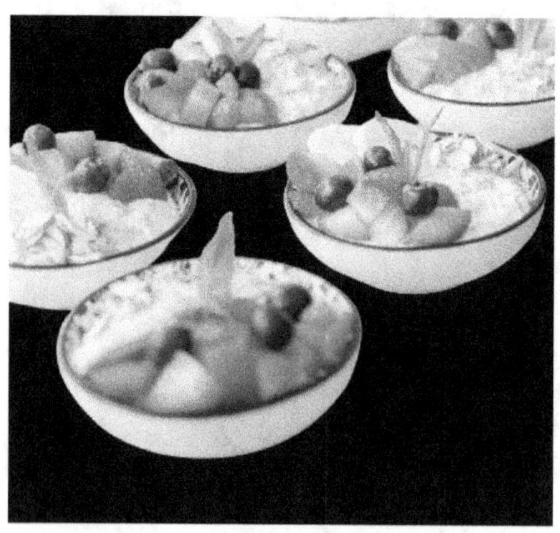

Chia Seed Pudding: Mix chia seeds with your choice of milk (such as almond, coconut, or cow's milk) and sweetener (like honey or agave syrup) in a jar or container. Let it sit in the refrigerator overnight to thicken. In the morning, top with fresh fruit, nuts, or coconut flakes for a nutritious and filling breakfast option.

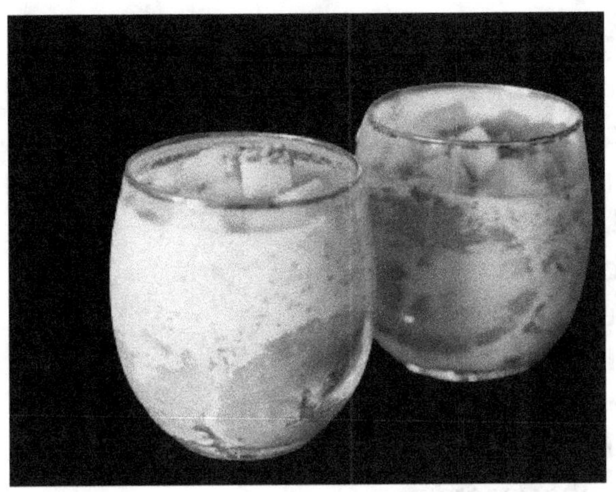

Overnight Oats Three Ways

Overnight oats are a versatile and convenient breakfast option that can be prepared in advance and customized to suit individual tastes. Here's how to make overnight oats three ways:

Traditional Overnight Oats: Components: half a cup of rolled oats
Half a cup of milk (vegan or dairy)
one-fourth cup Greek yogurt
One tablespoon of optional chia seeds
One tablespoon of maple syrup or honey (optional)
Guidelines:
Rollin oats, milk, Greek yogurt, chia seeds, and sweetener (if using) should all be combined in a jar or other container.
For all ingredients to be dispersed equally, give it a good stir.

Refrigerate the jar or container for at least four hours, preferably overnight. Cover it.
Stir the oats in the morning and top with your preferred toppings, like almond butter, seeds, nuts, or fresh fruit.

Ingredients for Chocolate Peanut Butter Overnight Oats:
Half a cup of rolled oats
Half a cup of milk (vegan or dairy)
one-fourth cup Greek yogurt
One tablespoon of optional chia seeds
One tsp of cocoa powder
One tablespoon of peanut butter
One tablespoon of maple syrup or honey (optional)
Guidelines:
Rollin oats, milk, Greek yogurt, chia seeds, cocoa powder, peanut butter, and sweetener (if using) should all be combined in a jar or other container.

Stir thoroughly to ensure that all ingredients are combined equally.

For at least four hours, preferably overnight, cover and chill.

Stir the oats in the morning and garnish with chopped peanuts, sliced bananas, and chocolate sauce for a decadent touch.

Ingredients for Berry Almond Overnight Oats:

Half a cup of rolled oats

Half a cup almond milk, or any other type of milk

one-fourth cup Greek yogurt

One tablespoon of optional chia seeds

1/4 cup of berries, including blueberries, raspberries, and strawberries

One spoonful of butter made of almonds

One tablespoon of maple syrup or honey (optional)

Guidelines:
Rollin oats, almond milk, Greek yogurt, chia seeds, mixed berries, almond butter, and sweetener (if needed) should all be combined in a jar or other container.
Blend until thoroughly blended.
For at least four hours, preferably overnight, cover and chill.
For an extra taste and crunch in the morning, toss in some more berries, cut almonds, and sprinkle some honey over the oats.

Veggie Egg Muffins

Veggie egg muffins are a nutritious and convenient breakfast option that can be prepared in advance and enjoyed throughout the week. Here's how to make them:

Ingredients:
6 large eggs
1/4 cup milk (dairy or plant-based)
Salt and pepper, to taste
1 cup diced vegetables (such as bell peppers, spinach, onions, tomatoes, mushrooms, or broccoli)
1/2 cup shredded cheese (optional)
Cooking spray or olive oil for greasing muffin tin.

Instructions:
Preheat the Oven: Preheat your oven to 350°F (175°C) and grease a 12-cup muffin tin with cooking spray or olive oil.

Prepare the Vegetables: Wash and chop your choice of vegetables into small, bite-sized pieces. You can use a variety of vegetables or whatever you have on hand.

Whisk the Eggs: In a large mixing bowl, whisk together the eggs, milk, salt, and pepper until well combined. The milk helps make the egg muffins light and fluffy.

Add the Vegetables: Stir the diced vegetables into the egg mixture until evenly distributed. You can also add shredded cheese at this stage if desired, for added flavor and creaminess.

Fill the Muffin Tin: Pour the egg and vegetable mixture evenly into the prepared muffin tin, filling each cup about 3/4 full. Use a spoon to distribute the vegetables evenly.

To bake the egg muffins, preheat the oven to 20 to 25 degrees Celsius. Bake the muffins until the tops are gently golden and the center of the muffins is set. A toothpick can be used to test the doneness of muffins; if it comes out clean, the muffins are done.

Cool and Store: Remove the egg muffins from the oven and allow them to cool in the muffin tin for a few minutes before carefully removing them with a spatula. Transfer the egg muffins to a wire rack to cool completely before storing.

Store and Reheat: Once cooled, store the egg muffins in an airtight container in the refrigerator for up to 5 days. To reheat, simply microwave them for 30-60 seconds until warmed through.

Veggie egg muffins are a versatile breakfast option that can be customized with your favorite vegetables, herbs, and spices. They're packed with protein, fiber, and essential nutrients, making them a healthy and satisfying way to start your day. Plus, they're portable and perfect for meal prep, making busy mornings a breeze.

Quinoa Breakfast Bowl

Quinoa breakfast bowls are a nutritious and filling option for a healthy meal prep breakfast. Here's how to make them:

Ingredients:
1 cup quinoa
2 cups water or vegetable broth
Pinch of salt
Your choice of toppings, such as:
Fresh fruit (berries, sliced bananas, diced mango)
Nuts and seeds (almonds, walnuts, chia seeds)
Greek yogurt or coconut yogurt
Honey or maple syrup
Nut butter (almond butter, peanut butter)
Cinnamon or other spices
Dried fruit (raisins, cranberries)
Coconut flakes

Instructions:
Rinse the Quinoa: Rinse the quinoa under cold water in a fine mesh strainer to remove any bitterness. Drain well.

Cook the Quinoa: In a saucepan, combine the rinsed quinoa with water or vegetable broth and a pinch of salt. Bring to a boil over medium-high heat, then reduce the heat to low, cover, and simmer for about 15 minutes, or until the quinoa is cooked and the liquid is absorbed. Remove from heat and let it sit, covered, for 5 minutes.

Fluff the Quinoa: After resting, uncover the saucepan and fluff the quinoa with a fork to separate the grains. Allow it to cool slightly before portioning it into individual containers for meal prep.

Prepare Toppings: While the quinoa is cooking, prepare your choice of toppings. Wash and slice any fresh fruit, toast nuts and seeds if desired, and portion out any additional ingredients you plan to add to your breakfast bowls.

Assemble Breakfast Bowls: To assemble each breakfast bowl, spoon a portion of cooked quinoa into a bowl or container. Top with your desired toppings, such as fresh fruit, nuts, seeds, yogurt, honey, or nut butter.

Store and Serve: Once assembled, cover the breakfast bowls with lids or plastic wrap and store them in the refrigerator for up to 4-5 days. When ready to eat, simply remove a bowl from the refrigerator, give it a stir, and enjoy cold or warm it up in the microwave for a few seconds before serving.

Chia Seed Pudding

Chia seed pudding is a nutritious and delicious option for healthy meal prep, especially for breakfast or as a snack. Here's how to make it:

One-fourth cup of chia seeds
One cup of your preferred milk (vegan or dairy)
Your preferred sweetener, such as agave syrup, maple syrup, or honey (optional)
Toppers or flavorings, including chocolate powder, vanilla essence, fresh fruit, nuts, or seeds (optional).

Instructions:
Mix Chia Seeds and Milk: In a bowl or jar, combine the chia seeds and milk. Stir well to evenly distribute the chia seeds in the milk. If desired, add sweetener to taste and any flavorings such as vanilla extract or cocoa powder.

Let it Set: Cover the bowl or jar and refrigerate the mixture for at least 4 hours, or preferably overnight. During this time, the chia seeds will absorb the liquid and swell, creating a thick, pudding-like consistency.

Stir and Serve: After the chia seed pudding has set, give it a good stir to ensure the seeds are evenly distributed and the pudding is smooth. At this point, you can taste and adjust the sweetness or add additional flavorings if desired.

Add Toppings: Before serving, garnish the chia seed pudding with your favorite toppings. Fresh fruit, such as berries or sliced bananas, adds natural sweetness and texture. Nuts, seeds, coconut flakes, or a drizzle of nut butter can also be delicious additions for added flavor and crunch.

Store for Meal Prep: Chia seed pudding can be stored in an airtight container in the refrigerator for up to 4-5 days, making it perfect for meal prep. Portion the pudding into individual containers or jars for easy grab-and-go breakfasts or snacks throughout the week.

Chia seed pudding is a nutrient-dense food, rich in fiber, protein, and omega-3 fatty acids. It's also naturally gluten-free and can be customized to suit various dietary preferences and tastes. Whether enjoyed plain or with a variety of toppings, chia seed pudding is a satisfying and nourishing option for healthy meal prep.

CHAPTER THREE

Lunch Recipes

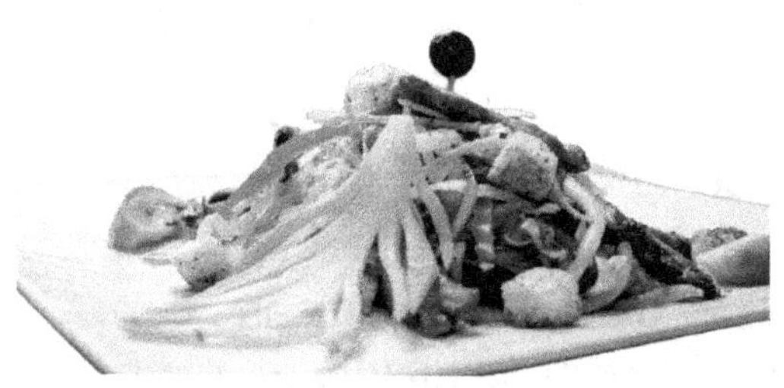

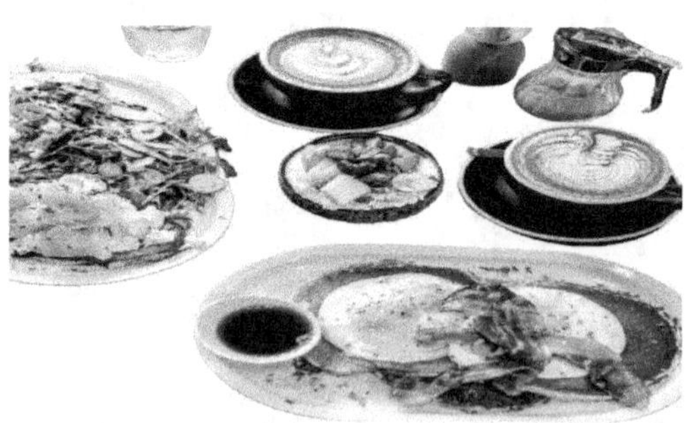

Here are some lunch recipes suitable for healthy meal prep:

Quinoa salad with vegetables and chickpeas:
As directed on the package, prepare the quinoa and allow it to cool.
Cooked quinoa, rinsed and drained chickpeas, diced veggies (bell peppers, cucumbers, cherry tomatoes, and red onions), and chopped fresh herbs (parsley or cilantro) should all be combined in a big bowl.
Use a basic vinaigrette composed of olive oil, lemon juice, garlic, salt, and pepper to dress the salad.
Scoop the salad into separate bowls for a filling and healthy lunch choice.

Chicken and Vegetable Stir-Fry:
Cut chicken breast into bite-sized pieces and marinate with soy sauce, ginger, garlic, and a touch of honey.
Stir-fry the marinated chicken in a skillet until cooked through, then remove from the pan and set aside.
In the same skillet, stir-fry a variety of chopped vegetables (such as bell peppers, broccoli, snap peas, carrots, and mushrooms) until crisp-tender.
Return the cooked chicken to the skillet and toss everything together with a splash of low-sodium soy sauce or teriyaki sauce.
Portion the stir-fry into meal prep containers and serve with cooked brown rice or quinoa for a balanced and flavorful lunch.

Mason Jar Salads:
Layer mason jars with your favorite salad
ingredients, starting with dressing at the
bottom, followed by hearty ingredients like
grains or proteins, and finishing with delicate
greens on top to prevent them from getting
soggy.
Choose a variety of colorful vegetables, leafy
greens, proteins (such as grilled chicken, tofu,
or hard-boiled eggs), nuts, seeds, and cheese.
Seal the jars tightly and store them in the
refrigerator until ready to eat. When you're
ready to enjoy, shake the jar to distribute the
dressing evenly and pour the salad onto a
plate or bowl.

Spread mashed avocado on a whole wheat or
spinach tortilla to make a turkey and avocado
wrap.

Arrange the sliced turkey breast, cucumber,
tomato, lettuce, and any additional fillings you
choose on top of the avocado.
Tuck the sides in as you carefully roll up the
tortilla.
For a well-balanced and easily transportable
lunch, cut the wrap in half and place it in a
lunchbox with some fresh fruit, baby carrots, or
whole grain crackers.

Make a base of cooked quinoa, brown rice, or
mixed greens for your vegetarian Buddha bowl.
Add a variety of steamed or roasted veggies
(kale, sweet potatoes, Brussels sprouts, and
cauliflower) on top.
For satiety, include protein foods like tempeh,
tofu, or chickpeas.
Drizzle with a tasty dressing or condiment, like
peanut sauce, tahini, or balsamic vinaigrette.
For extra taste and texture, garnish with
toasted nuts or seeds, avocado slices, and
fresh herbs.

Chicken and Veggie Stir-Fry

Chicken and veggie stir-fry is a delicious and nutritious meal that can be prepared ahead of time for healthy meal prep. Here's how to make it:

Ingredients:
2 boneless, skinless chicken breasts, thinly sliced
2 cups mixed vegetables (such as bell peppers, broccoli, snap peas, carrots, and mushrooms), chopped
2 cloves garlic, minced
1 tablespoon ginger, grated or minced
2 tablespoons low-sodium soy sauce or tamari
1 tablespoon sesame oil
1 tablespoon olive oil or vegetable oil
Salt and pepper, to taste
Cooked brown rice or quinoa, for serving.

Instructions:

Marinate the Chicken: In a bowl, combine the thinly sliced chicken breast with minced garlic, grated ginger, and low-sodium soy sauce. Toss well to coat the chicken evenly in the marinade. Let it marinate for at least 15-20 minutes, or up to overnight in the refrigerator for maximum flavor.

Prepare the Vegetables: While the chicken is marinating, wash and chop your choice of mixed vegetables into bite-sized pieces. You can use a variety of colorful vegetables to add flavor, texture, and nutrients to the stir-fry.

To stir-fry the chicken, place a large skillet or wok over medium-high heat and add olive or vegetable oil. When the oil is hot, place the marinated chicken slices in a single layer in the skillet.

Cook the chicken for two to three minutes on each side, or until it is cooked through and browned. After taking the chicken out of the skillet, set it aside.

Cook the Vegetables: In the same skillet, add a little more oil if needed, then add the chopped vegetables. Stir-fry the vegetables for 4-5 minutes, or until they are crisp-tender and slightly caramelized.

Combine Chicken and Vegetables: Return the cooked chicken to the skillet with the vegetables. Stir well to combine and heat through, allowing the flavors to meld together.

Season and Serve: Drizzle the stir-fry with sesame oil for added flavor and richness. Season with salt and pepper to taste, if needed. Serve the chicken and veggie stir-fry hot over cooked brown rice or quinoa for a complete and satisfying meal.

Meal Prep: Divide the chicken and veggie stir-fry into individual meal prep containers, along with a portion of cooked brown rice or quinoa. Let the containers cool completely before sealing and storing them in the refrigerator for up to 4-5 days.

Chicken and veggie stir-fry is a nutritious and versatile meal prep option that's packed with protein, fiber, vitamins, and minerals. It's a balanced meal that can be customized with your favorite vegetables and enjoyed for lunch or dinner throughout the week. Plus, it's quick and easy to make, making it perfect for busy weekdays.

Greek Salad in a Jar

Ingredients:
1/4 cup extra virgin olive oil
2 tablespoons red wine vinegar
1 tablespoon fresh lemon juice
1-2 cloves garlic, minced
1 teaspoon dried oregano
Salt and pepper to taste
1 cup chopped cucumber
1 cup halved cherry tomatoes
1/2 cup diced red onion
1/2 cup crumbled feta cheese
1/4 cup pitted Kalamata olives
2 cups chopped romaine lettuce or baby spinach.

Instructions:
Prepare the Dressing:
In a small bowl, whisk together the olive oil, red wine vinegar, lemon juice, minced garlic, dried oregano, salt, and pepper. Taste and adjust seasonings as needed.

Layer the Mason Jar:
Begin by pouring a couple of tablespoons of the prepared dressing into the bottom of a clean quart-sized mason jar.

Add Sturdy Ingredients:
Start layering the chopped cucumber, halved cherry tomatoes, and diced red onion on top of the dressing. These ingredients can withstand the dressing without becoming soggy.

Add Protein and Flavor:
Next, add layers of crumbled feta cheese and pitted Kalamata olives on top of the vegetables. If desired, you can also add sliced grilled chicken or chickpeas for extra protein.

Add Greens:
Finish off the layers with chopped romaine lettuce or baby spinach leaves. These greens will stay crisp and fresh until you're ready to eat.

Seal and Refrigerate:
Secure the lid tightly onto the mason jar and store it in the refrigerator. The salad will stay fresh for up to 4-5 days.

Serve and Enjoy:
When you're ready to eat, give the jar a good shake to distribute the dressing evenly. You can either eat the salad directly from the jar or transfer it to a bowl. Enjoy your delicious and nutritious Greek Salad on the go!

Tips:
Make sure to pack the ingredients tightly in the jar to prevent air from getting in, which can cause the salad to wilt faster.
Feel free to customize the ingredients based on your preferences. You can add or omit ingredients like bell peppers, artichoke hearts, or grilled shrimp.

Keep the dressing separate if you prefer to add it just before eating to maintain maximum freshness.
Store the mason jars upright in the refrigerator to prevent the dressing from leaking out.
Consider making several jars at once for easy grab-and-go lunches throughout the week.

Turkey and Avocado Wraps

Ingredients:
4 large whole wheat or spinach tortillas
1 ripe avocado, sliced
8 slices of deli turkey
1 cup shredded lettuce or baby spinach
1/2 cup shredded cheese (cheddar, Monterey
Jack, or your choice)
1/4 cup diced tomatoes
1/4 cup diced red onion (optional)
1/4 cup sliced black olives (optional)
1/4 cup Greek yogurt or mayonnaise
Salt and pepper to taste

Instructions:
Prepare the Ingredients:
Slice the avocado, dice the tomatoes, red
onion (if using), and slice the black olives (if
using).

Assemble the Wraps:
Lay out the tortillas on a clean surface.
Spread a thin layer of Greek yogurt or
mayonnaise evenly over each tortilla.
Place two slices of deli turkey onto each tortilla,
leaving a border around the edges.
Layer the sliced avocado, shredded lettuce or
baby spinach, diced tomatoes, diced red onion
(if using), and sliced black olives (if using)
evenly over the turkey.

Season and Add Cheese:
Sprinkle salt and pepper to taste over the
fillings.
Sprinkle shredded cheese evenly over each
wrap.

Roll the Wraps:
Starting from one end, tightly roll up each
tortilla, tucking in the edges as you go to
prevent the fillings from falling out.

Slice and Serve:
Use a sharp knife to slice each wrap in half
diagonally or into smaller pinwheel slices.
Serve immediately, or wrap each wrap tightly in
plastic wrap or foil for later enjoyment.

Tips:
Feel free to customize the wraps with your
favorite ingredients such as sliced bell
peppers, shredded carrots, or hummus.
To make it spicy, you can add a dash of hot
sauce or sprinkle red pepper flakes over the
fillings.
If preparing ahead of time, store the wraps in
an airtight container in the refrigerator for up to
24 hours to keep them fresh.
These wraps are perfect for a quick lunch,
snack, or light dinner.

Buddha Bowl Varieties

Buddha bowls are vibrant, nourishing meals typically composed of a variety of vegetables, grains, proteins, and dressings, all served in a bowl. They are not only visually appealing but also packed with nutrients, making them an excellent option for healthy meal prep. Here are some common Buddha bowl varieties and components:

Base: Start with a nutrient-rich base such as quinoa, brown rice, barley, or couscous. These whole grains provide complex carbohydrates, fiber, and essential nutrients.

Protein: Add a source of protein to your Buddha bowl to help keep you feeling satisfied and to support muscle repair and growth. Options include grilled chicken, tofu, tempeh, chickpeas, black beans, lentils, or edamame.

Vegetables: Fill your bowl with an assortment of colorful vegetables to provide an array of vitamins, minerals, and antioxidants. Examples include leafy greens (spinach, kale), bell peppers, broccoli, carrots, cucumbers, tomatoes, roasted sweet potatoes, and avocado.

Healthy fats: Incorporate sources of healthy fats to promote satiety and support overall health. Avocado slices, nuts (such as almonds, walnuts, or cashews), seeds (like pumpkin seeds or sesame seeds), or a drizzle of olive oil or tahini can be excellent choices.

Flavorful additions: Enhance the flavor of your Buddha bowl with herbs, spices, and condiments. Fresh herbs like cilantro, parsley, or basil can add brightness, while spices such as cumin, turmeric, paprika, or garlic powder can add depth. Hummus, salsa, pesto, or a homemade vinaigrette can also elevate the taste of your bowl.

Optional extras: Feel free to customize your Buddha bowl with additional ingredients based on your preferences and dietary needs. This could include roasted seaweed, kimchi, pickled vegetables, grilled fruit (such as pineapple or mango), or a sprinkle of nutritional yeast for added umami flavor.

By incorporating a variety of ingredients into your Buddha bowls, you can create endless combinations that are not only delicious but also provide a balanced and nutritious meal. Plus, by preparing components in advance, such as cooking grains and proteins and chopping vegetables, you can streamline the meal prep process for quick and easy assembly throughout the week.

CHAPTER FOUR

Dinner Recipes

Healthy dinner recipes for meal prep are a great way to ensure you have nutritious and delicious meals ready to go throughout the week. Here are some ideas for dinner recipes that are perfect for meal prep:

Sheet Pan Chicken and Vegetables: Season chicken breasts with your favorite herbs and spices, then roast them alongside a variety of colorful vegetables like bell peppers, broccoli, and sweet potatoes on a sheet pan. Divide into meal prep containers and pair with a side of quinoa or brown rice for a balanced meal.

Stir-fry a variety of your favorite veggies, including broccoli, carrots, bell peppers, and snap peas, with tofu cubes in a tasty sauce made with soy sauce, ginger, garlic, and a dash of honey or maple syrup. Serve with cooked quinoa or brown rice for a filling supper choice.

Turkey and Quinoa Stuffed Bell Peppers: Fill halved bell peppers with a mixture of cooked quinoa, lean ground turkey, black beans, corn, diced tomatoes, and spices. Bake until the peppers are tender and the filling is heated through. These stuffed peppers can be portioned out for easy reheating during the week.

Salmon and Asparagus Foil Packets: Season salmon filets with lemon juice, garlic, and herbs, then place them on a sheet of foil along with asparagus spears.

Seal the packets tightly and bake until the salmon is cooked through and the asparagus is tender. Serve with a side of roasted potatoes or a mixed green salad.

Chickpea and Vegetable Curry: Simmer chickpeas, diced vegetables (such as cauliflower, carrots, and bell peppers), and spinach in a flavorful curry sauce made from coconut milk, curry paste, and spices like turmeric, cumin, and coriander. Serve over cooked brown rice or quinoa for a satisfying and comforting meal.

Mason Jar Salads: Layer mason jars with your favorite salad ingredients such as mixed greens, cherry tomatoes, cucumbers, shredded carrots, chickpeas, and grilled chicken or tofu. Keep the dressing separate until ready to eat to prevent the salad from getting soggy. These portable salads are perfect for on-the-go dinners.

Quinoa and Black Bean Enchilada Casserole: Layer cooked quinoa, black beans, diced bell peppers, onions, and enchilada sauce in a baking dish. Top with shredded cheese (or a dairy-free alternative) and bake until bubbly. Divide into portions and serve with a side of avocado slices and salsa.

Mediterranean Chicken Bowls: Marinate chicken breasts in lemon juice, olive oil, garlic, and Mediterranean herbs like oregano and thyme. Grill or bake until cooked through, then slice. Serve over a bed of mixed greens and quinoa, and add toppings like cherry tomatoes, cucumber slices, olives, and feta cheese. Drizzle with a balsamic vinaigrette before serving.

Vegetable Lentil Soup: Simmer lentils, diced tomatoes, carrots, celery, onions, and vegetable broth in a large pot until the lentils are tender and the vegetables are cooked through.

Season with herbs like thyme, rosemary, and bay leaves for flavor. Portion into containers for easy reheating throughout the week, and serve with a side of crusty whole grain bread.

Thai Peanut Tofu Bowls: Marinate tofu cubes in a mixture of peanut butter, soy sauce, lime juice, garlic, and ginger. Bake until golden and crispy. Serve over cooked brown rice or rice noodles, and add sautéed vegetables like bell peppers, broccoli, and snap peas. Garnish with chopped peanuts, cilantro, and a squeeze of lime for freshness.

One-Pan Baked Salmon with Roasted Vegetables

One-Pan Baked Salmon with Roasted Vegetables is a convenient and nutritious meal prep option that requires minimal effort and cleanup. Here's how to make it:

Ingredients:
Salmon filets
Assorted vegetables (such as broccoli, bell peppers, carrots, and zucchini)
Olive oil
Garlic powder
Paprika
Salt and pepper
Lemon wedges (optional, for serving)
Instructions:
Preheat the oven: Preheat your oven to 400°F (200°C) and line a large baking sheet with parchment paper or aluminum foil for easy cleanup.

Get the veggies ready: After washing, cut the veggies you've selected into bite-sized pieces. Place them on one side of the baking sheet that has been prepared in a single layer.

Season the vegetables: Drizzle the vegetables with olive oil and sprinkle with garlic powder, paprika, salt, and pepper to taste. Toss them gently to coat evenly.

Prepare the salmon: Place the salmon filets on the other side of the baking sheet, leaving some space between each filet. Drizzle the salmon with olive oil and season with salt, pepper, and a sprinkle of garlic powder.

Bake: Transfer the baking sheet to the preheated oven and bake for 12-15 minutes, or until the salmon is cooked through and flakes easily with a fork, and the vegetables are tender and lightly browned.

Serve or portion for meal prep: Once cooked, remove the baking sheet from the oven. Serve the salmon and vegetables immediately with lemon wedges for squeezing over the salmon, if desired. Alternatively, let the meal cool slightly before portioning it into meal prep containers for easy reheating throughout the week.

Advice: Feel free to alter this dish by adding your preferred vegetables or by adding alternative herbs and spices to the salmon. When you're ready to cook, just put everything on the baking sheet after chopping the veggies and seasoning the salmon, to save time.
Any leftovers can be kept for up to three or four days in the refrigerator in an airtight container. Before serving, reheat in the oven or microwave until well heated.
Not only is this one-pan meal delicious and healthful, but it's also ideal for hectic weeknights when you need a filling and speedy supper choice.

Lentil and Vegetable Curry

Lentil and Vegetable Curry is a flavorful and nutritious dish that's perfect for meal prep. Here's how to make it:

Ingredients:

1 cup dried lentils (any variety)

2 tablespoons olive oil or coconut oil

1 onion, diced

3 cloves garlic, minced

1 tablespoon grated ginger

2 carrots, diced

2 potatoes, diced

1 bell pepper, diced

1 zucchini, diced

1 can (14 oz) diced tomatoes

1 can (14 oz) coconut milk

2 tablespoons curry powder

1 teaspoon ground turmeric

1 teaspoon ground cumin

1 teaspoon ground coriander

Salt and pepper to taste

Fresh cilantro for garnish (optional)

Cooked rice or naan bread for serving.

Guidelines:
Prepare the lentils: After giving the lentils a quick rinse in cold water, transfer them to a pot and add just enough water to cover by approximately one inch. After bringing to a boil, lower the heat, and simmer the lentils for 20 to 25 minutes, or until they are soft but not falling apart. After draining, leave the cooked lentils aside.

To prepare the veggies, heat the olive oil in a large pot or Dutch oven over medium heat. Cook for approximately five minutes, or until the diced onion is tender. Cook for an additional minute or until aromatic after adding the grated ginger and minced garlic.

Add the vegetables: Add the diced carrots, potatoes, bell pepper, and zucchini to the pot. Cook for 5-7 minutes, stirring occasionally, until the vegetables begin to soften.

Make the curry: Stir in the diced tomatoes, coconut milk, curry powder, turmeric, cumin, coriander, salt, and pepper. Bring the mixture to a simmer, then reduce the heat to low and let it simmer for 15-20 minutes, or until the vegetables are tender and the flavors have melded together.

Add the cooked lentils: Stir the cooked lentils into the curry mixture, and let it simmer for another 5-10 minutes to heat through and allow the flavors to blend.

Serve: Taste and adjust the seasoning if necessary. Serve the lentil and vegetable curry hot, garnished with fresh cilantro if desired, and accompanied by cooked rice or naan bread.

Advice: This curry is great for meal prep because it can be prepared in advance and kept in the fridge for up to 4-5 days.
You can certainly alter the vegetables to suit your tastes or what you have on hand.
You can add some diced chili pepper or a dash of cayenne pepper to the pot with the other spices if you want your curry hotter.
You may reheat leftover curry in the microwave or on the stovetop until it's well heated.
Savor this filling and wholesome lentil and vegetable curry as a tasty and productive weeknight dinner prep alternative!

Stuffed Bell Peppers

A tasty and adaptable dish that's ideal for healthy meal planning is stuffed bell peppers. This is how to prepare them:

Four sizable bell peppers, any color will do
One cup of cooked rice or quinoa
One can (15 oz) of rinsed and drained black beans
One cup of fresh, frozen, or canned corn kernels
one cup of tomatoes, chopped
One little onion, chopped finely
two minced garlic cloves
One teaspoon of cumin powder
One tsp of chili powder
To taste, add salt and pepper.
One cup of shredded cheese, such as Monterey Jack, cheddar, or a dairy-free substitute
For garnish, use fresh parsley or cilantro (optional).

Guidelines:
Warm up the oven: Turn the oven on to 375°F, or 190°C. Grease a baking dish that is big enough to accommodate the upright bell peppers.

Cut off the tops of the bell peppers and remove the seeds and membranes from within to prepare them. Remove a small coating from the bottom of each pepper if necessary so that they stand straight in the baking dish. After the baking dish is ready, put the peppers inside.

To make the filling, put the cooked rice or quinoa, black beans, corn, diced tomatoes, onion, garlic, ground cumin, chili powder, salt, and pepper in a large mixing bowl. Mix thoroughly until fully incorporated.

Fill the peppers: Using a spoon, carefully spoon the filling mixture into each bell pepper until it reaches the top. In order to pack the filling inside, gently press down. Top each stuffed pepper with shredded cheese, if you'd like.

Bake: Cover the baking dish with foil and bake in the preheated oven for 30-35 minutes, or until the peppers are tender and the filling is heated through. If using cheese, remove the foil during the last 10 minutes of baking to allow the cheese to melt and lightly brown.

Serve: Remove the stuffed bell peppers from the oven and let them cool for a few minutes before serving. Garnish with fresh cilantro or parsley if desired.

Advice: You can alter the filling to suit your tastes. For extra protein, try adding diced cooked chicken or ground turkey. For extra nutrition, add chopped spinach or kale.

For up to three to four days, leftover stuffed bell peppers can be kept in the refrigerator in an airtight container. Before serving, reheat them in the oven or microwave until well heated.

For extended storage, stuffed bell peppers can also be frozen. After cooling down individually, cover each pepper in foil and plastic wrap before putting it in a freezer bag. Before heating, let it thaw in the fridge for the entire night.

Savor these mouthwatering stuffed bell peppers for a filling and healthy lunch or dinner alternative!

Teriyaki Tofu Stir-Fry

This tasty, high-protein dish, Teriyaki Tofu Stir-Fry, is ideal for making nutritious meal prep. This is how to prepare it:

Ingredients: 1 block (14 oz) diced and pressed firm tofu
Two teaspoons of vegetable or sesame oil
Two cups of sliced mixed veggies (carrots, bell peppers, broccoli, snap peas, and mushrooms)
three minced garlic cloves
One tablespoon of finely chopped ginger
1/4 cup tamari or low-sodium soy sauce
two tsp of rice vinegar
Two tablespoons of maple syrup or honey
One tablespoon of cornflour
two tsp water
Prepared quinoa or rice for serving
As a garnish, add chopped green onions and sesame seeds (optional).

Instructions:
Press and prepare the tofu: Wrap the block of tofu in paper towels or a clean kitchen towel and place a heavy object on top (such as a cast iron skillet or a couple of cans). Let it sit for 15-30 minutes to press out excess moisture. Then, cut the tofu into cubes.

Prepare the sauce: In a small bowl, whisk together the soy sauce, rice vinegar, honey or maple syrup, minced garlic, and grated ginger.

To cook the tofu, place a large skillet or wok over medium-high heat with one tablespoon of oil. Add the tofu cubes and heat for 5 to 7 minutes, or until brown and crispy on all sides. After taking the tofu out of the skillet, set it aside.

Stir-fry the vegetables: Pour the remaining tablespoon of oil into the same skillet. When the mixed vegetables are crisp-tender, add them to the skillet and stir-fry for 4–5 minutes.

Reintroduce the cooked tofu to the skillet along with the vegetables, then cover everything with the teriyaki sauce. To ensure even coating, stir.

To thicken the sauce, slurry-make the cornstarch and water in a small bowl. Stir thoroughly after adding the slurry to the skillet. Simmer the sauce for an additional one to two minutes, or until it thickens.

Serve: Top cooked rice or quinoa with the hot teriyaki tofu stir-fry. If desired, garnish with chopped green onions and sesame seeds.

Advice: Feel free to alter the vegetables to suit your tastes or what you have on hand.

Sliced onions, diced bell peppers, or sliced mushrooms can be added to the stir-fry to add more flavor.

Stir-fry leftovers keep well in the refrigerator for three to four days when kept in an airtight container. Before serving, reheat it in a skillet or microwave until thoroughly warmed.

To make this a gluten-free version, substitute tamari for the soy sauce.

Savor this tasty and wholesome Teriyaki Tofu Stir-Fry for a filling lunch or dinner alternative!

CHAPTER FIVE

Snacks and Sides

When it comes to healthy meal prep, snacks and sides are essential for keeping you satisfied between meals and adding variety to your meals. Here are some ideas for healthy snacks and sides you can prep in advance:

Snacks:
Vegetable Sticks with Hummus: Pre-cut carrots, cucumber, bell peppers, and celery sticks and portion them into individual containers. Pair with small containers of hummus for a satisfying and nutritious snack.

Greek Yogurt Parfaits: Layer Greek yogurt with fresh berries, sliced bananas, and a sprinkle of granola or nuts in small jars or containers. These parfaits are rich in protein, calcium, and fiber.

Trail Mix: Make your own trail mix by combining nuts (such as almonds, walnuts, or cashews), seeds (like pumpkin seeds or sunflower seeds), and dried fruits (such as raisins, cranberries, or apricots). Portion out into small bags or containers for a convenient grab-and-go snack.

Hard-Boiled Eggs: Cook a batch of hard-boiled eggs and store them in the refrigerator for a quick and protein-rich snack. Sprinkle it with a little salt and pepper or your favorite seasoning blend for added flavor.

Homemade Energy Balls: Mix together ingredients like rolled oats, nut butter, honey or maple syrup, and add-ins like chocolate chips, chia seeds, or shredded coconut. Roll into bite-sized balls and store them in the refrigerator for a convenient energy boost.

Sides:
Roasted Vegetables: Chop up a variety of vegetables (such as broccoli, cauliflower, carrots, and Brussels sprouts), toss them with olive oil and your favorite herbs and spices, and roast them in the oven until tender and caramelized. These make a delicious and colorful side dish for any meal.

Quinoa Salad: Cook a batch of quinoa and mix it with chopped vegetables (like cucumbers, tomatoes, and bell peppers), fresh herbs (such as parsley or cilantro), and a simple vinaigrette dressing. This salad is hearty, nutritious, and can be served cold or at room temperature.

Steamed Greens: Steam leafy greens like spinach, kale, or Swiss chard and toss them with a squeeze of lemon juice and a drizzle of olive oil. Season with salt and pepper to taste a simple and healthy side.

Stuffed Bell Peppers: Make a batch of stuffed bell peppers filled with a mixture of cooked quinoa or rice, black beans, corn, diced tomatoes, and spices. These make a satisfying side dish or light meal.

Cucumber Salad: Slice cucumbers thinly and toss them with red onion, cherry tomatoes, feta cheese, and a light vinaigrette dressing for a refreshing and crunchy side salad.

By prepping these snacks and sides in advance, you'll have healthy options readily available to enjoy throughout the week, making mealtime convenient and nutritious.

Energy Bites

Energy bites are bite-sized snacks packed with nutritious ingredients that provide a quick burst of energy. They are perfect for healthy meal prep because they're easy to make, portable, and can be customized to suit your taste preferences. Here's how to make energy bites:

Ingredients:
1 cup rolled oats
1/2 cup nut butter (such as almond butter, peanut butter, or cashew butter)
1/4 cup honey or maple syrup
1/4 cup ground flaxseed or chia seeds
1/4 cup unsweetened shredded coconut
1/4 cup mini chocolate chips or dried fruit (optional)
1 teaspoon vanilla extract
Pinch of salt.

Instructions:

Combine ingredients: In a large mixing bowl, combine rolled oats, nut butter, honey or maple syrup, ground flaxseed or chia seeds, shredded coconut, chocolate chips or dried fruit (if using), vanilla extract, and a pinch of salt. Stir until well combined.

Chill mixture: Place the mixture in the refrigerator for 15-30 minutes to firm up slightly. Chilling the mixture makes it easier to roll into balls.

Roll into balls: After the mixture has cold, take small quantities and roll them into bite-sized balls using your hands or a spoon. They are customizable to your desired size.

Store: Place the energy bites on a baking sheet lined with parchment paper and refrigerate for at least 1 hour to set. Once set, transfer them to an airtight container and store them in the refrigerator for up to 1 week, or in the freezer for longer storage.

Tips:
Customize your energy bites by adding different mix-ins such as chopped nuts, seeds, dried fruit, cocoa powder, or spices like cinnamon or nutmeg.
If the mixture is too dry, add a little more nut butter or honey/maple syrup. If it's too wet, add more oats or flaxseed/chia seeds to bind it together.
Energy bites are versatile and can be enjoyed as a quick snack, pre-workout fuel, or even a healthy dessert.

Pack a few energy bites in your lunchbox or gym bag for a convenient on-the-go snack that will keep you energized and satisfied throughout the day.
By making a batch of energy bites during your meal prep session, you'll have a nutritious and delicious snack ready whenever you need a quick pick-me-up.

Hummus and Veggie Sticks

Hummus and veggie sticks make for a delicious and nutritious snack that's perfect for healthy meal prep. Here's how to prepare them:

Ingredients:
1 cup cooked chickpeas (or 1 can, drained and rinsed)
2 tablespoons tahini
2 tablespoons lemon juice
1 clove garlic, minced
2 tablespoons olive oil
Salt and pepper to taste
Assorted vegetables for dipping (carrot sticks, cucumber slices, bell pepper strips, celery sticks, cherry tomatoes, etc.)

Instructions:

Prepare the hummus: In a food processor, combine the cooked chickpeas, tahini, lemon juice, minced garlic, olive oil, salt, and pepper. Blend until smooth and creamy, adding a splash of water if needed to reach your desired consistency.

Taste and adjust: Taste the hummus and adjust the seasoning if necessary. You can add more lemon juice, garlic, salt, or tahini to suit your preferences.

Prepare the vegetables: Wash and cut assorted vegetables into sticks, slices, or bite-sized pieces. Arrange them on a plate or in individual containers for easy snacking.

Serve: Transfer the hummus to a serving bowl and place it alongside the prepared vegetable sticks. Optionally, drizzle a little extra olive oil on top of the hummus and sprinkle with paprika or chopped fresh herbs for garnish.

Store: If you're preparing these for meal prep, portion the hummus into individual containers and pack them alongside the vegetable sticks. Store them in the refrigerator for up to 4-5 days.

Tips:
Feel free to customize your hummus by adding additional ingredients such as roasted red peppers, sun-dried tomatoes, fresh herbs (like parsley or cilantro), or spices (like cumin or paprika).
For extra flavor and texture, sprinkle toasted sesame seeds, pine nuts, or dukkah (a Middle Eastern spice blend) on top of the hummus before serving.

To keep the vegetables crisp, you can store them in a separate container lined with a paper towel to absorb excess moisture.

Hummus and veggie sticks are not only a great snack but also make a healthy addition to lunchboxes, party platters, or picnics.

Enjoy this simple and nutritious snack of hummus and veggie sticks as a convenient option for healthy meal prep!

Roasted Chickpeas Three Ways

Roasted chickpeas are a crunchy and flavorful snack that can be seasoned in a variety of ways. Here are three different seasoning options for roasted chickpeas:

Standard Roasted Chickpeas: Components:
One can (15 oz) of washed, drained, and patted dry chickpeas
One tablespoon of olive oil
To taste, add salt and pepper.
Guidelines:
Set oven temperature to 400°F, or 200°C.
Toss the chickpeas with olive oil in a bowl until they are well coated.
Arrange the chickpeas evenly on a parchment paper-lined baking sheet.
Roast the chickpeas for 20 to 30 minutes in a preheated oven, stirring the pan from time to time, until they are crispy and golden brown.
To taste, add salt and pepper for seasoning.
Before serving, allow to cool.

Spicy Roasted Chickpeas:
Ingredients:
1 can (15 oz) chickpeas, drained, rinsed, and patted dry
1 tablespoon olive oil
1 teaspoon chili powder
1/2 teaspoon paprika
1/2 teaspoon cumin
Salt to taste
Instructions:
Preheat your oven to 400°F (200°C).
In a bowl, toss the chickpeas with olive oil until evenly coated.
Sprinkle the chili powder, paprika, cumin, and salt over the chickpeas and toss to coat.
Arrange the chickpeas evenly on a parchment paper-lined baking sheet.
Roast the chickpeas for 20 to 30 minutes in a preheated oven, stirring the pan from time to time, until they are crispy and golden brown.
Before serving, allow to cool.

Sweet and Spicy Roasted Chickpeas:
Ingredients:
1 can (15 oz) chickpeas, drained, rinsed, and
patted dry
1 tablespoon olive oil
1 tablespoon honey or maple syrup
1/2 teaspoon cinnamon
1/4 teaspoon cayenne pepper
Salt to taste
Instructions:
Preheat your oven to 400°F (200°C).
In a bowl, toss the chickpeas with olive oil until
evenly coated.
Drizzle the honey or maple syrup over the
chickpeas and sprinkle with cinnamon,
cayenne pepper, and salt. Toss to coat.
Arrange the chickpeas evenly on a parchment
paper-lined baking sheet.
Roast the chickpeas for 20 to 30 minutes in a
preheated oven, stirring the pan from time to
time, until they are crispy and golden brown.
Before serving, allow to cool.

Guacamole and Whole Grain Crackers

Guacamole and whole grain crackers make for a delicious and satisfying snack or appetizer. Here's how to prepare them:

Ingredients for guacamole: two ripe avocados
One little tomato, chopped
1/4 cup of coarsely chopped red onion
one minced garlic clove
One tablespoon of lime juice
One tablespoon of freshly cut cilantro
To taste, add salt and pepper.
Guidelines:
Remove the pits from the avocados, cut them in half, and scoop the flesh into a mixing bowl. Using a fork, mash the avocado until it's smooth, or leave it chunky if you'd rather. Add the diced tomato, chopped red onion, minced garlic, lime juice, chopped cilantro, salt, and pepper to the mashed avocado. Stir until well combined.

Taste and adjust the seasoning if necessary.
Add more lime juice, salt, or pepper to suit your
taste.
Transfer the guacamole to a serving bowl and
garnish with additional chopped cilantro or a
sprinkle of paprika if desired.
Serve immediately with whole grain crackers
for dipping, or cover and refrigerate until ready
to serve.

Complete Grain Crackers:
Components:
One cup of flour made from whole wheat
Half a cup of rolled or quick oats
one-fourth cup of sesame seeds
one-fourth cup of sunflower seeds
1/4 cup of flaxseeds
one-fourth cup olive oil
one-fourth cup water
Half a teaspoon each of salt and optional garlic
powder
Half a teaspoon powdered onion, optional.

Guidelines:

Adjust the oven temperature to 350°F (175°C) and place parchment paper on a baking pan.

The whole wheat flour, oats, sesame seeds, sunflower seeds, flaxseeds, salt, garlic powder, and onion powder (if used) should all be combined in a sizable mixing basin.

Mix the dry ingredients with the water and olive oil until a dough forms. One tablespoon at a time, add extra water to the dough if it's too dry until it comes together.

On a surface dusted with flour, roll out the dough to a thickness of about 1/8 inch.

The dough can be cut into squares or rectangles using a pizza cutter or a sharp knife.

Place the crackers onto the baking sheet that has been prepared, and bake for 15 to 20 minutes, or until crisp and golden brown.

Before serving, take the crackers out of the oven and allow them to cool fully.
Serving suggestions: Place the bowl of guacamole and the whole grain crackers on a dish or serving tray. Serve as a tasty and wholesome appetizer or snack for any occasion.

CHAPTER SIX

Desserts

Desserts don't have to be skipped during healthy meal planning! By choosing desserts that are produced with healthful ingredients and have less added sugar, you may still enjoy sweets while adhering to your dietary goals. The following dessert ideas are ideal for a healthy dinner prep:

Fruit Salad:
Prepare a colorful fruit salad using a variety of fresh fruits such as berries, melons, grapes, kiwi, and pineapple.
Optionally, toss the fruit with a squeeze of lemon or lime juice to keep it fresh and vibrant.
Portion the fruit salad into individual containers for easy grab-and-go desserts throughout the week.

Greek Yogurt Parfaits:
Layer Greek yogurt with fresh berries, sliced
bananas, and a sprinkle of granola or chopped
nuts.
Greek yogurt is high in protein and calcium,
making it a nutritious base for a satisfying
dessert.
Portion the parfaits into jars or containers and
store them in the refrigerator for a quick and
easy dessert option.

Chia Seed Pudding:
Mix chia seeds with your choice of milk (such
as almond milk, coconut milk, or dairy milk)
and a touch of sweetener (such as honey,
maple syrup, or agave nectar).
Let the mixture sit in the refrigerator for a few
hours or overnight until thickened.
Serve the chia seed pudding topped with fresh
fruit, nuts, or coconut flakes for added flavor
and texture.

Spread Greek yogurt onto a baking sheet that has been coated with parchment paper to make frozen yogurt bark.
Add sliced fruit, nuts, seeds, and a drizzle of honey or melted dark chocolate to the yogurt's surface.
For a tasty and cool frozen treat, freeze the bark until solid, then break it into pieces.

Baked Fruit Crisp:
Make a fruit crisp using a combination of your favorite fruits (such as apples, berries, peaches, or pears) topped with a mixture of oats, whole wheat flour, nuts, and a touch of sweetener.
Bake until the fruit is bubbling and the topping is golden brown and crispy.
Serve the fruit crisp warm or at room temperature, optionally with a dollop of Greek yogurt or a scoop of vanilla ice cream.

Dark Chocolate Covered Fruit:
Dip fresh fruit (such as strawberries, banana slices, or orange segments) into melted dark chocolate.
Place the chocolate-covered fruit on a baking sheet lined with parchment paper and refrigerate until the chocolate is set.
Enjoy the sweet and indulgent treat in moderation as a satisfying dessert option.

These dessert ideas are not only delicious but also nutritious, providing you with vitamins, minerals, and fiber while satisfying your sweet tooth. Prepare them in advance during your meal prep session to have healthier dessert options readily available throughout the week.

Fruit Salad with Honey-Lime Dressing

Fruit salad with honey-lime dressing is a refreshing and flavorful dessert that's perfect for healthy meal prep. Here's how to make it:

Ingredients:
For the fruit salad:
Assorted fresh fruits (such as strawberries, blueberries, raspberries, blackberries, grapes, kiwi, pineapple, mango, and/or oranges), washed, peeled, and chopped as needed
For the honey-lime dressing:
2 tablespoons honey
Juice of 1 lime
Zest of 1 lime
1 tablespoon chopped fresh mint or basil (optional).

Instructions:
Prepare the fruit: Wash and chop the assorted fruits as needed and place them in a large mixing bowl. You can use any combination of fruits you like, depending on your preferences and what's in season.

Make the dressing: In a small bowl, whisk together the honey, lime juice, and lime zest until well combined. If desired, add chopped fresh mint or basil for an extra burst of flavor.

Toss the fruit with the dressing: Pour the honey-lime dressing over the chopped fruit in the mixing bowl. Gently toss until all the fruit is evenly coated with the dressing.

Chill: Cover the fruit salad with plastic wrap or transfer it to an airtight container and refrigerate for at least 30 minutes to allow the flavors to meld together and the fruit to chill.

Serve: When ready to serve, give the fruit salad a final toss to redistribute the dressing. Optionally, garnish with additional fresh mint or basil leaves for presentation.

Enjoy: Serve the fruit salad with honey-lime dressing as a refreshing and nutritious dessert option. It's perfect for serving at gatherings, potlucks, or simply as a sweet treat after a meal.

Tips:
Feel free to customize the fruit salad with your favorite fruits or whatever is in season. You can also add a handful of nuts or seeds for added crunch and protein.
To suit your taste, add more or less honey to the dressing to change its sweetness.
For optimal results, be sure to utilize ripe and flavorful fruits.

To make an eye-catching fruit salad, you can also combine various textures and hues.
You may refrigerate leftover fruit salad for up to two or three days if you keep it in an airtight container. Just remember that some fruits could leak their juices over time, so mix it gently each time you serve it.
Savor this colorful and flavorful fruit salad with a honey-lime dressing for a nutritious and revitalizing dessert choice!

Dark Chocolate Bark with Nuts and Seeds

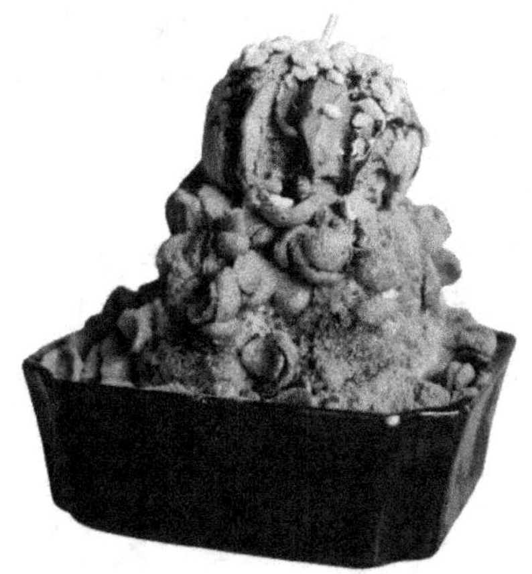

Dark chocolate bark with nuts and seeds is a delicious and satisfying dessert that's perfect for healthy meal prep. Here's how to make it:

Ingredients:
8 ounces dark chocolate (at least 70% cocoa), chopped
1/2 cup mixed nuts (such as almonds, walnuts, cashews, or pistachios), roughly chopped

1/4 cup mixed seeds (such as pumpkin seeds, sunflower seeds, or sesame seeds)
Flaky sea salt, for sprinkling (optional).

Guidelines:
Get a baking sheet ready: Place a silicone baking mat or parchment paper on a baking sheet and set it aside.

To melt chocolate, put chopped dark chocolate in a bowl that is safe to put in the microwave. Heat the chocolate in the microwave for 30 second bursts, stirring in between, until it melts and becomes smooth. As an alternative, you can use a double boiler to melt the chocolate.

Spread the chocolate: Pour the melted chocolate onto the prepared baking sheet and use a spatula to spread it out into an even layer, about 1/4-inch thick.

Add the nuts and seeds: Sprinkle the chopped nuts and mixed seeds evenly over the melted chocolate, pressing them down slightly so they adhere to the chocolate.

Sprinkle with sea salt: If desired, sprinkle a small amount of flaky sea salt over the top of the chocolate bark for a sweet and salty flavor contrast.

Chill: Place the baking sheet in the refrigerator for about 30 minutes, or until the chocolate is set and firm.

Break into pieces: Once the chocolate bark is completely set, remove it from the refrigerator and break it into pieces using your hands or a knife.

Store: Store the dark chocolate bark with nuts and seeds in an airtight container in the refrigerator for up to 1-2 weeks. Alternatively, you can store it in the freezer for longer storage.

Tips:
Choose dark chocolate with at least 70%
cocoa content for a rich and intense flavor.
Dark chocolate is also higher in antioxidants
and lower in sugar compared to milk chocolate.
Feel free to customize the bark by adding dried
fruit, coconut flakes, or spices like cinnamon or
chili powder for extra flavor.
For a smoother texture, you can temper the
chocolate before spreading it on the baking
sheet. Tempering helps to ensure that the
chocolate sets properly and has a glossy finish.
Serve the dark chocolate bark with nuts and
seeds as a delicious and satisfying dessert or
snack. It's also a great homemade gift idea for
special occasions.
Enjoy this indulgent yet nutritious dark
chocolate bark with nuts and seeds as a
guilt-free treat during your healthy meal prep!

Banana Nice Cream

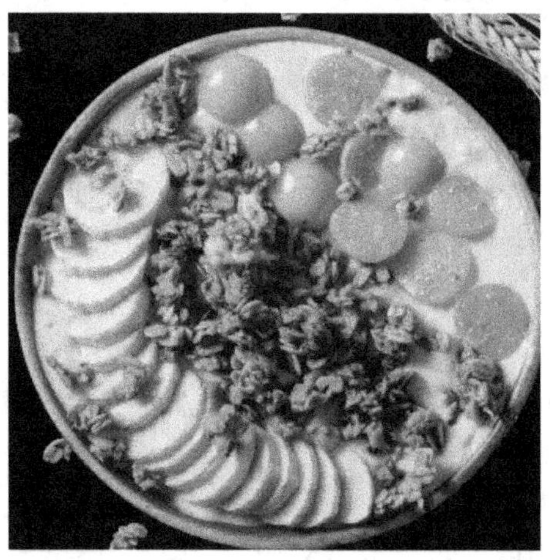

Banana nice cream is a healthy and delicious alternative to traditional ice cream, made with just one ingredient – bananas! Here's how to make it:

Ingredients:
Ripe bananas, peeled and sliced (use as many bananas as you'd like, depending on how much nice cream you want to make)
Optional add-ins and toppings:
Vanilla extract
Cocoa powder
Peanut butter or almond butter
Frozen berries or other fruits
Nuts (such as almonds, walnuts, or pecans)
Chocolate chips
Coconut flakes
Honey or maple syrup for added sweetness.

Guidelines:
Get the bananas ready: After the bananas are ripe, peel and cut them into coins. Place the banana slices in a single layer on a parchment paper-lined baking sheet. Verify that the slices are not in contact with one another.

Freeze the bananas: Place the baking sheet in the freezer and freeze the banana slices for at least 2-3 hours, or until they are completely frozen.

Blend the bananas: Once the banana slices are frozen solid, transfer them to a blender or food processor. Blend the bananas on high speed until smooth and creamy, stopping to scrape down the sides of the blender or food processor as needed. You may need to add a splash of milk or dairy-free milk alternative to help the blending process.

Add optional ingredients: If desired, add any optional add-ins such as vanilla extract, cocoa powder, peanut butter, frozen berries, or other fruits to the blender and blend until combined.

Serve: Transfer the banana nice cream to serving bowls or cones. Optionally, sprinkle with your favorite toppings such as nuts, chocolate chips, coconut flakes, or a drizzle of honey or maple syrup.

Enjoy immediately: Banana nice cream is best enjoyed immediately while it's still creamy and soft. If you have any leftovers, you can transfer them to an airtight container and store them in the freezer for later. However, keep in mind that the texture may become harder after freezing, so you may need to let it soften at room temperature for a few minutes before serving.

Advice: Ripe bananas yield the maximum sweetness and flavor. Additionally, ripe bananas will mix into a creamy texture more readily.

Try varying the flavors by adding your preferred ingredients, such as frozen berries for a fruity touch, peanut butter for a nutty flavor, or cocoa powder for chocolate lovely cream.
You can combine the frozen banana slices with a small amount of milk or a dairy-free milk substitute to get a creamier consistency if you'd have a softer texture.
Savor this rich and smooth banana lovely cream as a guilt-free snack or dessert while preparing your nutritious meals!

Baked Apple Slices with Cinnamon

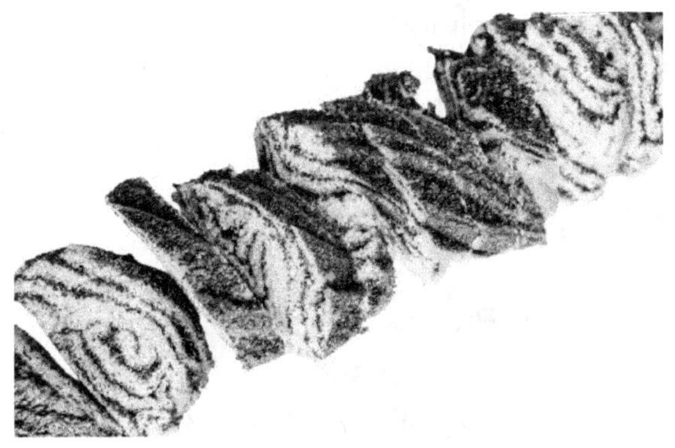

Baked apple slices with cinnamon are a warm and comforting dessert that's simple to make and perfect for healthy meal prep. Here's how to make them:

Ingredients:
4 medium apples (such as Granny Smith, Honeycrisp, or Gala)
1 tablespoon lemon juice
1 tablespoon honey or maple syrup (optional)
1 teaspoon ground cinnamon
Pinch of nutmeg (optional)
Pinch of salt
Instructions:
Preheat the oven: Preheat your oven to 375°F (190°C) and line a baking sheet with parchment paper or lightly grease it with cooking spray.

Prepare the apples: Wash the apples and slice them into thin rounds, about 1/4-inch thick. You can leave the peel on or peel the apples, depending on your preference. Remove the cores and seeds from the apple slices.

Toss with lemon juice: Place the apple slices in a large mixing bowl and toss them with lemon juice to prevent them from browning.

Season the apples: In a small bowl, mix together the honey or maple syrup (if using), ground cinnamon, nutmeg (if using), and salt. Sprinkle the cinnamon mixture over the apple slices and toss to coat evenly.

Arrange on baking sheet: Spread the seasoned apple slices out in a single layer on the prepared baking sheet. Make sure the slices are not overlapping to ensure even baking.

Bake: Transfer the baking sheet to the preheated oven and bake the apple slices for 15-20 minutes, or until they are tender and lightly golden brown around the edges.

Serve: Remove the baked apple slices from the oven and let them cool slightly before serving. You can enjoy them warm or at room temperature.

Optional toppings: Serve the baked apple slices with a dollop of Greek yogurt, a sprinkle of granola, or a drizzle of honey or maple syrup for added sweetness.

Tips:

Feel free to customize the seasoning of the baked apple slices according to your taste preferences. You can add a pinch of ground cloves or ginger for extra warmth and flavor. Serve the baked apple slices on their own as a simple and healthy dessert, or use them as a topping for oatmeal, yogurt, or pancakes. Leftover baked apple slices can be stored in an airtight container in the refrigerator for up to 3-4 days. Reheat them in the microwave or enjoy them cold as a quick and easy snack. Enjoy these warm and fragrant baked apple slices with cinnamon as a cozy and nutritious dessert option during your healthy meal prep!

CHAPTER SEVEN

Drinks and Smoothies

Drinks and smoothies can be excellent additions to a healthy meal prep routine, providing hydration, nutrients, and even a boost of energy. Here's a comprehensive overview:

Hydration:
Water: The most essential drink for hydration. Infusing water with fruits or herbs can add flavor without extra calories or sugar.
Herbal teas: Calorie-free options like green tea or herbal blends can provide hydration along with antioxidants and other health benefits.

Smoothies:

Base: Start with a liquid base such as water, milk (dairy or plant-based), or yogurt. These provide hydration, protein, and calcium.

Fruits: Add a variety of fruits for vitamins, minerals, and natural sweetness. Berries, bananas, mangoes, and pineapple are popular choices.

Vegetables: Sneak in some veggies like spinach, kale, or cucumber for added nutrients and fiber.

Protein: Include protein sources like protein powder, Greek yogurt, or silken tofu to keep you feeling full and support muscle repair and growth.

Healthy fats: Add sources like avocado, nuts, or seeds for heart-healthy fats that promote satiety.

Flavor boosters: Enhance the flavor with ingredients like honey, cinnamon, ginger, or cocoa powder.

Ice: For a refreshing texture, add ice cubes or frozen fruits.

Benefits of Drinks and Smoothies in Meal Prep:

Convenience: Preparing drinks and smoothies in advance saves time during busy mornings or as grab-and-go options.

Nutrient density: By including a variety of fruits, vegetables, proteins, and healthy fats, drinks and smoothies can pack a powerful nutritional punch.

Portion control: Preparing drinks and smoothies in advance allows for portion control and ensures you're getting the right balance of nutrients.

Customization: Tailor drinks and smoothies to your taste preferences and dietary needs, whether you're vegan, gluten-free, or have specific health goals.

Healthy Advice: Pay attention to portion sizes and added sugars, particularly those found in fruit juices, yogurts, and syrups that have been sweetened.

To ensure a diversity of nutrients and to keep things interesting, try experimenting with different food combinations.

To cut down on waste, think about storing drinks and smoothies in mason jars or reusable water bottles.

Use items that provide extra fiber and omega-3 fatty acids, such as flaxseeds or chia seeds.

You may support your overall health and wellness goals and keep nourished, hydrated, and energetic throughout the day by including beverages and smoothies in your meal prep routine.

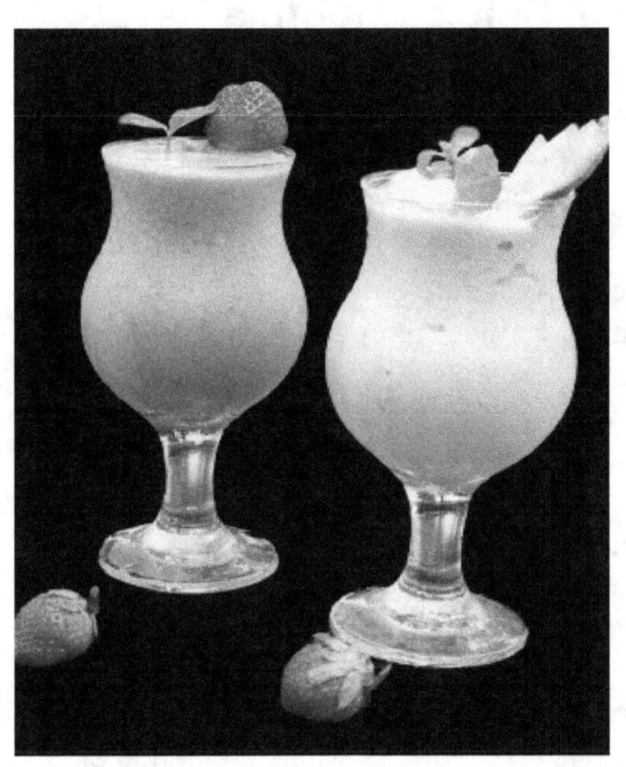

Green Detox Smoothie

A nutrient-rich drink called a green detox smoothie is intended to help nourish and cleanse the body. Here's how to get it ready for a nutritious meal prep:

Ingredients: Leafy greens (Swiss chard, spinach, or kale are great options). Rich in vitamins, minerals, and antioxidants, these greens promote general health and detoxification.

Liquid base: Use water, coconut water, almond milk, or another liquid of your choice as the base of the smoothie.

Fruits: Add sweetness and additional nutrients with fruits like bananas, apples, pineapple, or mango. These fruits provide natural sugars and fiber.

Vegetables: Enhance the detoxifying properties of the smoothie with vegetables like cucumber, celery, or parsley. These veggies are hydrating and contain compounds that support liver function and detoxification.

Protein: Include a protein source such as Greek yogurt, protein powder, or hemp seeds to make the smoothie more satisfying and support muscle repair and growth.

Healthy fats: Incorporate ingredients like avocado, chia seeds, or flaxseeds for added healthy fats, fiber, and omega-3 fatty acids.

Flavor enhancers: Add lemon juice, ginger, or mint leaves for extra flavor and detoxifying benefits.

Instructions:
Prep ingredients: Wash and chop the leafy greens, fruits, and vegetables as needed.

Blend: In a blender, combine the leafy greens, fruits, vegetables, protein source, healthy fats, and flavor enhancers. Add the liquid base to achieve your desired consistency.

Blend until smooth: Start the blender on low speed and gradually increase to high until all ingredients are well blended and smooth.

Taste and adjust: Taste the smoothie and adjust the sweetness or flavor as needed by adding more fruits or flavor enhancers.

Store: Pour the smoothie into individual serving containers or mason jars with lids for easy grab-and-go options during your meal prep.

Healthy Tips:

Experiment with different combinations of ingredients to find your favorite Green Detox Smoothie recipe.

Use organic ingredients when possible to minimize exposure to pesticides and other harmful chemicals.

Drink the smoothie fresh for maximum nutritional benefits, but it can also be stored in the refrigerator for up to 24 hours.

Consider adding a scoop of green superfood powder for an extra boost of nutrients and detoxification support.

Berry Blast Smoothie

A Berry Blast Smoothie is a delicious and nutritious beverage packed with the goodness of berries. Here's how to prepare it for healthy meal prep:

Ingredients:
Berries: Choose a variety of berries such as strawberries, blueberries, raspberries, and blackberries. Berries are rich in antioxidants, vitamins, and fiber, making them excellent for overall health and immune support.

Liquid base: Use water, coconut water, almond milk, or another liquid of your choice as the base of the smoothie.

Banana: Adding a ripe banana helps to sweeten the smoothie naturally and provides a creamy texture. Bananas also offer potassium and other essential nutrients.

Greek yogurt: Greek yogurt adds creaminess, protein, and probiotics to the smoothie, promoting gut health and helping you feel full and satisfied.

Protein powder (optional): You may choose to add a scoop of protein powder to your smoothie to make it higher in protein. Select a premium protein powder that fits your dietary requirements.

Flavor enhancers: Enhance the flavor of the smoothie with ingredients like honey, vanilla extract, or a squeeze of lemon juice.

Instructions:

Prep ingredients: Wash the berries and remove any stems or hulls. Peel and slice the banana if needed.

Blend: In a blender, combine the berries, banana, Greek yogurt, protein powder (if using), flavor enhancers, and liquid base.

Blend until smooth: Start the blender on low speed and gradually increase to high until all ingredients are well blended and smooth.

Taste and adjust: Taste the smoothie and adjust the sweetness or flavor as needed by adding more honey, vanilla extract, or lemon juice.

Store: Pour the smoothie into individual serving containers or mason jars with lids for easy grab-and-go options during your meal prep.

Healthy Tips:
Experiment with different combinations of
berries to find your favorite flavor profile.
Consider adding a handful of spinach or kale
for an extra boost of nutrients and greens.
Use frozen berries for a thicker and colder
smoothie, or add ice cubes if using fresh
berries.
If you're watching your sugar intake, skip the
honey and rely on the natural sweetness of the
berries and banana.

By incorporating a Berry Blast Smoothie into
your healthy meal prep routine, you can enjoy
a refreshing and nutritious beverage that
provides a burst of flavor and essential
nutrients to fuel your day.

Ginger Turmeric Lemonade

Ginger Turmeric Lemonade is a refreshing and immune-boosting beverage known for its anti-inflammatory properties and zesty flavor. Here's how to prepare it for healthy meal prep:

Ingredients:
Turmeric root or powder: Turmeric is renowned for its anti-inflammatory and antioxidant properties. You can use fresh turmeric root (peeled and sliced) or ground turmeric powder.

Ginger root: Ginger adds a spicy kick and additional anti-inflammatory benefits to the lemonade. Use fresh ginger root (peeled and sliced) for the best flavor.

Lemon: Freshly squeezed lemon juice provides a tangy flavor and a boost of vitamin C. You'll need several lemons depending on the desired tartness.

Honey or maple syrup: These natural sweeteners offer a hint of sweetness and temper the acidity of the lemon. Adapt the quantity to your personal taste preferences.

Water: Use filtered water to make the base of the lemonade.

Instructions:
Prepare ingredients: Wash and peel the turmeric and ginger roots if using fresh. Slice them into thin rounds or grate them for easier blending.

Make turmeric-ginger base: In a blender, combine the turmeric, ginger, and a small amount of water. Blend until smooth to create a concentrated turmeric-ginger paste.

Make lemonade: In a large pitcher, combine the turmeric-ginger paste, freshly squeezed lemon juice, honey or maple syrup, and the remaining water. Stir well to combine.

Taste and adjust: Taste the lemonade and adjust the sweetness or tartness by adding more honey, lemon juice, or water as needed.

Store: Transfer the ginger turmeric lemonade into individual serving containers or airtight jars with lids for easy storage during your meal prep.

Healthy Tips:
You can customize the flavor by adding additional ingredients like mint leaves or a pinch of black pepper for enhanced absorption of turmeric's active compound, curcumin.
To save time, you can make a larger batch of the turmeric-ginger paste and store it in the refrigerator for up to a week. Then, simply mix it with lemon juice, honey, and water whenever you want to prepare a fresh batch of lemonade. Enjoy the ginger turmeric lemonade chilled over ice for a refreshing drink, or warm it up for a soothing beverage during colder months.
Be cautious with turmeric, as it can stain surfaces and clothing easily. Wash any utensils, countertops, or cutting boards immediately after use.

Incorporating Ginger Turmeric Lemonade into your healthy meal prep routine can provide a flavorful and health-boosting beverage option to support your overall well-being.

Iced Herbal Tea Recipes

Iced herbal tea recipes are refreshing, hydrating, and packed with health benefits. Here's how to prepare them for healthy meal prep:

Ingredients:
Herbal tea bags: Choose your favorite herbal tea blends such as chamomile, peppermint, hibiscus, rooibos, or a combination of herbs. Opt for organic tea bags for the best quality and flavor.

Water: Use filtered water to brew the tea.

Optional flavorings: Enhance the flavor of your iced herbal tea with ingredients like fresh citrus slices (lemon, lime, or orange), herbs (mint, basil, or lavender), spices (cinnamon sticks or ginger slices), or natural sweeteners (honey, agave syrup, or stevia).

Ice: To chill the tea and create a refreshing iced beverage.

Instructions:
Brew the tea: Bring a pot of water to a boil and remove it from heat. Add the herbal tea bags to the hot water and steep according to the package instructions, usually 5-10 minutes depending on the type of herbal tea and desired strength.

Sweeten (if desired): You can taste-test and add natural sweeteners like honey, agave syrup, or stevia while the tea is still warm. Until the sweetener is completely dissolved, stir.

Cool the tea: Allow the brewed tea to cool to room temperature before transferring it to the refrigerator to chill for at least 1-2 hours or until completely cold.

Add flavorings: Once the tea is chilled, you can add additional flavorings to enhance the taste. Experiment with citrus slices, herbs, spices, or other natural flavorings. Let the tea infuse with these ingredients for a few hours in the refrigerator for optimal flavor.

Serve: Fill glasses with ice cubes and pour the chilled herbal tea over the ice. Garnish with additional citrus slices, herbs, or spices if desired.

Store: If you're preparing the iced herbal tea in advance for meal prep, store it in airtight containers or glass bottles in the refrigerator for up to 2-3 days. Shake or stir well before serving.

Healthy Tips:
Herbal teas are caffeine-free and rich in antioxidants, making them a healthy alternative to sugary beverages.

Experiment with different herbal tea blends and flavor combinations to keep things interesting.
To reduce waste, use reusable tea bags or loose-leaf herbal teas with a tea infuser.
Avoid adding excessive amounts of sweeteners to keep the drink as healthy as possible.
Feel free to adjust the strength of the tea and the amount of ice based on your personal preference for flavor and temperature.

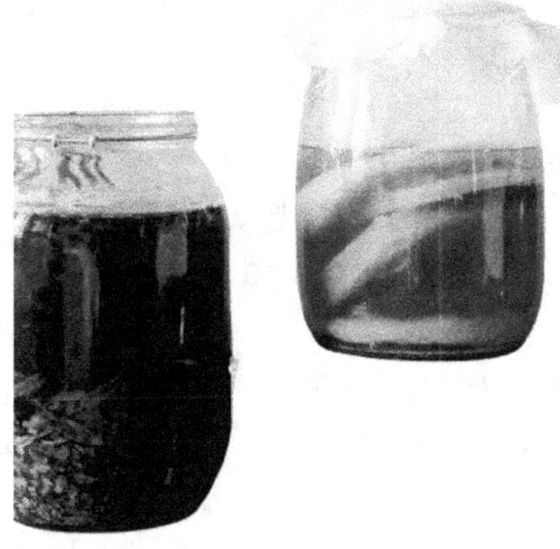

CHAPTER EIGHT

Special Dietary Needs

Healthy meal prep can accommodate various special dietary needs to ensure that individuals with specific dietary restrictions or preferences can still enjoy nutritious and satisfying meals. Here's an overview of some common special dietary needs and considerations for healthy meal prep:

Vegetarianism and Veganism:
Vegetarian: Excludes meat, poultry, and seafood but may include dairy products and eggs.
Vegan: Excludes all animal products, including meat, poultry, seafood, dairy, eggs, and sometimes honey.

Meal prep options: Focus on plant-based proteins such as beans, lentils, tofu, tempeh, and seitan. Incorporate a variety of vegetables, fruits, whole grains, nuts, and seeds to ensure balanced nutrition.

Gluten-Free:
Avoids gluten-containing grains such as wheat, barley, rye, and their derivatives.
Meal prep options: Use naturally gluten-free grains like rice, quinoa, buckwheat, millet, and gluten-free oats. Choose gluten-free versions of pasta, bread, and other grain-based products. Pay attention to cross-contamination in cooking utensils and kitchen surfaces.

Dairy-Free:
Avoids dairy products like milk, cheese, yogurt, and butter.

Meal prep options: Use plant-based milk alternatives such as almond, coconut, soy, or oat milk. Substitute dairy-free cheese or yogurt made from nuts, seeds, or coconut. Incorporate sources of calcium and vitamin D from fortified plant-based foods or supplements.

Low-Carb or Keto:
Limits carbohydrate intake and emphasizes fats and protein.
Meal prep options: Include non-starchy vegetables, lean proteins (such as poultry, fish, tofu, and eggs), and healthy fats (such as avocados, nuts, seeds, and olive oil). Limit or avoid high-carb foods like grains, starchy vegetables, and sugary foods.

Paleo:
Emphasizes whole foods similar to those available to our pre-agricultural ancestors, including meat, fish, eggs, vegetables, fruits, nuts, and seeds.
Meal prep options: Focus on whole, unprocessed foods and avoid grains, legumes, and dairy. Include plenty of lean proteins, vegetables, fruits, nuts, and seeds.

Food Allergies and Intolerances:
Individuals may have allergies or intolerances to specific foods such as nuts, shellfish, soy, or eggs.
Meal prep options: Carefully read food labels and avoid allergens. Substitute allergenic ingredients with suitable alternatives. Practice safe food handling and prevent cross-contamination in the kitchen.

Specific Health Conditions:
Certain health conditions like diabetes, hypertension, or heart disease may require specific dietary modifications.
Meal prep options: Consult with a healthcare professional or registered dietitian to create meal plans tailored to individual health needs. Focus on nutrient-dense foods, portion control, and monitoring key nutrients like carbohydrates, sodium, and saturated fats.

When meal prepping for individuals with special dietary needs, it's essential to communicate openly, plan ahead, and be mindful of ingredient choices to ensure that everyone can enjoy delicious, nourishing meals that meet their unique dietary requirements.

Gluten-Free Meal Prep Ideas

Gluten-free meal prep focuses on excluding ingredients containing gluten, such as wheat, barley, rye, and their derivatives, to accommodate individuals with gluten sensitivities or celiac disease. Here are some gluten-free meal prep ideas for healthy and delicious options:

Grain Bowls:
Base: Use gluten-free grains like quinoa, rice (brown, white, or wild), buckwheat, millet, or gluten-free oats.
Protein: Add grilled chicken, tofu, tempeh, chickpeas, or beans for protein.
Vegetables: Include a variety of roasted or sautéed vegetables such as bell peppers, broccoli, carrots, zucchini, and spinach.
Sauce: Drizzle with gluten-free sauces or dressings like tahini, pesto, salsa, or homemade vinaigrettes.

Stir-Fries:
Protein: Choose lean protein sources like shrimp, beef, chicken, or tofu.
Vegetables: Stir-fry a colorful mix of vegetables such as bell peppers, snap peas, onions, mushrooms, and bok choy.
Sauce: Use gluten-free tamari or coconut aminos instead of soy sauce for flavor. Add garlic, ginger, and chili flakes for extra kick.

Salads:
Greens: Start with a base of leafy greens like spinach, kale, arugula, or mixed greens.
Protein: Top with grilled salmon, hard-boiled eggs, canned tuna, or sliced turkey.
Add-ins: Include gluten-free toppings like avocado, nuts, seeds, roasted vegetables, and fresh fruits.
Dressing: Make homemade gluten-free dressings using olive oil, vinegar, lemon juice, herbs, and spices.

Soups and Stews:
Base: Use gluten-free broth or stock as the base for soups and stews.
Protein: Add lean proteins such as chicken, turkey, beef, or lentils.
Vegetables: Incorporate a variety of vegetables like carrots, celery, onions, potatoes, and tomatoes.
Seasoning: Flavor with herbs, spices, and gluten-free seasonings like garlic powder, onion powder, and dried herbs.

Snack Boxes:
Protein: Include gluten-free protein sources like hard-boiled eggs, cheese, hummus, or Greek yogurt.
Vegetables: Pack raw vegetables like carrot sticks, cucumber slices, cherry tomatoes, and sugar snap peas.
Fruits: Add fresh fruits such as apple slices, berries, grapes, or orange segments.
Nuts and Seeds: Include gluten-free nuts and seeds like almonds, walnuts, pumpkin seeds, or sunflower seeds for healthy fats and crunch.

Baked Goods:
Gluten-Free Flours: Use gluten-free flours like almond flour, coconut flour, rice flour, or chickpea flour for baking.
Recipes: Prepare gluten-free baked goods such as muffins, pancakes, waffles, or bread using gluten-free ingredients.
Sweeteners: Use natural sweeteners like honey, maple syrup, or coconut sugar instead of refined sugars.

When meal prepping gluten-free meals, it's essential to check labels for hidden sources of gluten in processed foods and to use separate utensils and cooking surfaces to prevent cross-contamination. With careful planning and creativity, gluten-free meal prep can offer a diverse range of nutritious and satisfying options for those with gluten sensitivities.

Vegan and Vegetarian Options

Vegan and vegetarian options for healthy meal prep focus on plant-based ingredients to provide nutrients, flavor, and variety. Here are some ideas for each:

Vegan Options:

Protein Sources:
Legumes: Include beans, lentils, chickpeas, and peas in salads, soups, stews, and curries.
Tofu and Tempeh: Use these versatile soy-based products in stir-fries, sandwiches, wraps, and Buddha bowls.
Seitan: Made from wheat gluten, seitan is a high-protein meat substitute that can be used in stir-fries, sandwiches, and wraps.
Plant-Based Protein Powder: Add vegan protein powder to smoothies, oats, or baked goods for an extra protein boost.

Grains and Carbohydrates:
Quinoa, Brown Rice, and Wild Rice: Use these gluten-free grains as a base for grain bowls, salads, and stir-fries.
Whole Wheat and Gluten-Free Pasta: Make pasta salads, stir-fries, or casseroles with vegan pasta and sauces.
Oats: Prepare overnight oats, oatmeal bars, or granola for breakfast or snacks.

Vegetables and Fruits:
Incorporate a variety of colorful vegetables and fruits into meals for added vitamins, minerals, and antioxidants.
Roast vegetables for bowls, salads, or side dishes.
Use fruits in smoothies, salads, or as toppings for oats and yogurt.

Healthy Fats:
Avocado: Enjoy avocado slices on toast, salads, sandwiches, or as a topping for grain bowls.

Nuts and Seeds: Add almonds, walnuts, chia seeds, flaxseeds, or hemp seeds to smoothies, salads, oatmeal, or snacks.

Vegetarian Options:

Dairy and Eggs:
Incorporate dairy products like milk, yogurt, cheese, and butter into meals for added protein, calcium, and flavor.
Use eggs in omelets, frittatas, quiches, or egg muffins for a protein-rich breakfast or snack option.

Plant-Based Protein:
Include dairy-based protein sources like Greek yogurt or cottage cheese in meals for added protein and creaminess.
Incorporate eggs into dishes like salads, sandwiches, wraps, and casseroles.

Meal Ideas:
Vegetarian Chili: Make a hearty chili using beans, vegetables, tomatoes, and spices. Serve with rice or cornbread.
Veggie Stir-Fry: Stir-fry a mix of colorful vegetables with tofu or tempeh and your favorite sauce. Serve over rice or noodles.
Caprese Salad: Layer slices of fresh tomatoes, mozzarella cheese, and basil leaves. Drizzle with olive oil and balsamic glaze.
Chickpea Salad: Combine chickpeas with diced vegetables, herbs, lemon juice, and olive oil for a refreshing salad.

When meal prepping vegan and vegetarian meals, focus on incorporating a variety of plant-based foods to ensure you're getting a wide range of nutrients. Plan your meals ahead of time, batch cook when possible, and store portions in containers for easy grab-and-go options throughout the week.

Low-Carb and Keto-Friendly Recipes

Low-carb and keto-friendly recipes for healthy meal prep focus on reducing carbohydrates while increasing healthy fats and moderate protein intake. Here are some ideas for low-carb and keto-friendly meal prep:

Protein Options:
Chicken Breast: Season and bake or grill chicken breasts for a versatile protein option that can be added to salads, wraps, or stir-fries.

Salmon: Bake or grill salmon filets and portion them out for meals. Salmon is rich in omega-3 fatty acids and provides a healthy source of protein and fat.

Ground Turkey or Beef: Cook lean ground turkey or beef with herbs and spices for use in tacos, lettuce wraps, or stuffed peppers.

Tofu or Tempeh: Marinate and bake tofu or tempeh for plant-based protein options that can be added to salads, stir-fries, or Buddha bowls.

Vegetables:
Leafy Greens: Prepare a variety of leafy greens such as spinach, kale, or arugula for salads, sautés, or omelets.

Cruciferous Vegetables: Roast or sauté cruciferous vegetables like broccoli, cauliflower, or Brussels sprouts for a low-carb side dish or meal component.

Zucchini Noodles: Use a spiralizer to make zucchini noodles ("zoodles") as a low-carb alternative to pasta. Toss with pesto, marinara sauce, or stir-fried vegetables.

Bell Peppers: Stuff bell peppers with ground meat, cheese, and spices for a low-carb and keto-friendly meal option.

Healthy Fats:
Avocado: Add sliced avocado to salads, sandwiches, or wraps for a creamy texture and healthy fats.

Nuts and Seeds: Include almonds, walnuts, chia seeds, flaxseeds, or hemp seeds as toppings for salads, yogurt, or snacks.

Olive Oil: Use olive oil for cooking and dressing salads. It's rich in monounsaturated fats and adds flavor to dishes.

Coconut Milk: Use full-fat coconut milk in curries, soups, or smoothies for a creamy texture and a source of healthy fats.

Meal Ideas:
Chicken Caesar Salad: Toss grilled chicken breast slices with romaine lettuce, cherry tomatoes, Parmesan cheese, and Caesar dressing.

Salmon with Roasted Vegetables: Serve baked salmon filets with roasted broccoli, cauliflower, and carrots seasoned with olive oil and herbs.

Tofu Stir-Fry: Stir-fry tofu with bell peppers, snap peas, and broccoli in a soy ginger sauce. Serve over cauliflower rice.

Egg Muffins: Make egg muffins with eggs, spinach, bell peppers, and cheese. Bake in muffin tins for a portable and protein-rich breakfast option.

Dairy-Free Alternatives

Incorporating dairy-free alternatives into meal prep is essential for individuals who are lactose intolerant, have dairy allergies, follow a vegan lifestyle, or simply prefer to avoid dairy products. Here's how to utilize dairy-free alternatives in healthy meal prep:

Milk Alternatives:
Choose from a variety of dairy-free milk options such as almond milk, soy milk, coconut milk, oat milk, rice milk, or cashew milk.
Use these milk alternatives in smoothies, oatmeal, cereal, coffee, tea, and baking recipes.

Cheese Alternatives:
Explore dairy-free cheese options made from nuts (like cashews or almonds), soy, coconut oil, or tapioca starch.

Use dairy-free cheese in sandwiches, wraps,
salads, casseroles, pizzas, or as a topping for
nachos and tacos.

Yogurt Alternatives:
Opt for dairy-free yogurt made from coconut
milk, almond milk, soy milk, or oat milk.
Incorporate dairy-free yogurt into parfaits,
smoothie bowls, overnight oats, salad
dressings, or as a topping for savory dishes.

Butter Alternatives:
Substitute dairy butter with plant-based
margarine, coconut oil, avocado, or olive oil in
cooking, baking, and spreading on toast.
Use these butter alternatives in recipes for
sauces, sautéing vegetables, baking cookies,
muffins, or pancakes.

Cream Alternatives:
Use dairy-free options like coconut cream or cashew cream as substitutes for heavy cream or whipped cream in recipes for soups, sauces, desserts, or coffee drinks.

Ice Cream Alternatives:
Enjoy dairy-free ice cream made from coconut milk, almond milk, soy milk, or cashew milk as a delicious dessert option.
Look for dairy-free ice cream flavors and brands that suit your taste preferences and dietary needs.

Baking Ingredients:
Replace dairy milk with dairy-free milk alternatives in baking recipes for cakes, muffins, bread, cookies, and other baked goods.
Experiment with dairy-free alternatives for ingredients like sour cream, cream cheese, and condensed milk in baking and dessert recipes.

When meal prepping with dairy-free
alternatives, it's important to check labels to
ensure that the products are free from dairy
ingredients and potential allergens. Consider
batch cooking dairy-free recipes, portioning out
servings into containers, and storing them in
the refrigerator or freezer for easy grab-and-go
options throughout the week. With careful
planning and creativity, dairy-free meal prep
can provide nutritious and delicious options for
individuals with various dietary preferences
and needs.

Batch Cooking Techniques

Batch cooking is a meal prep technique that involves preparing large quantities of food in advance to be portioned out and enjoyed throughout the week. It saves time, reduces stress, and helps maintain healthy eating habits. Here's how to utilize batch cooking techniques for healthy meal prep:

Plan Your Meals:
Decide which meals you want to prepare for the week, including breakfast, lunch, dinner, and snacks.
Choose recipes that are suitable for batch cooking and that can be easily reheated or assembled when needed.

Make a Grocery List:
Based on your meal plan, create a comprehensive grocery list of ingredients you'll need for batch cooking.
Check your pantry and fridge to see what items you already have on hand and only purchase what you need.

Set Aside Time: Choose a day or period of the week to dedicate to batch cooking. This may occur on a non-peak day or over the weekend. Set out a few hours in your calendar to devote yourself entirely to dinner preparation.

Choose Your Recipes:
Select recipes that are suitable for batch cooking and that can be easily scaled up to make larger portions.
Look for recipes that can be cooked in bulk using one-pot or sheet pan methods to minimize cleanup.

Prep Ingredients:
Wash, peel, chop, and portion out ingredients in advance to streamline the cooking process. Pre-cook grains, beans, and proteins if needed to save time during batch cooking.

Cook in Batches:
Prepare large quantities of food in batches, focusing on one recipe at a time.
Utilize multiple pots, pans, and kitchen appliances to cook different components simultaneously.

Portion and Store:
Once the food is cooked, portion it out into individual containers or meal prep containers. Label containers with the name of the dish and the date it was prepared for easy identification. Store containers in the refrigerator or freezer depending on when you plan to consume them.

Reheat and Enjoy:
When ready to eat, simply reheat the pre-cooked meals in the microwave, oven, or stovetop.
Add fresh garnishes, sauces, or toppings as desired to enhance flavor and variety.

Rotate and Refresh:
Throughout the week, mix and match different pre-cooked components to create a variety of meals.

As you finish meals, replenish your batch cooking supply by cooking another round of meals.
Batch cooking allows you to maintain a healthy and balanced diet even during busy times. It provides convenience, saves money, reduces food waste, and ensures that you always have nutritious meals ready to enjoy.

Troubleshooting Common Issues

Troubleshooting common issues that may arise during healthy meal prep involves identifying challenges and finding solutions to ensure successful and stress-free meal preparation. Here are some common issues and ways to address them:

Lack of Time:
Issue: Feeling overwhelmed with meal prep due to a busy schedule.
Solution: Prioritize efficiency by choosing quick and easy recipes, utilizing batch cooking techniques, and prepping ingredients in advance.

Recipe Fatigue:

Issue: Getting bored with eating the same meals repeatedly.

Solution: Incorporate variety by experimenting with different recipes, cuisines, flavors, and ingredients. Rotate meals throughout the week to keep things interesting.

Ingredient Spoilage:

Issue: Fresh ingredients going bad before they can be used.

Solution: Plan meals based on perishability, prioritize using fresh ingredients early in the week, and freeze or preserve ingredients that won't be used immediately. Properly store ingredients in the refrigerator or freezer to prolong their shelf life.

Overcooking or Undercooking:

Issue: Difficulty achieving the right level of doneness when cooking meals in advance.

Solution: Use kitchen tools like timers, thermometers, and recipe guidelines to ensure accurate cooking times and temperatures. Practice cooking techniques to improve consistency.

Taste and Flavor:
Issue: Meals tasting bland or unappetizing.
Solution: Enhance flavor by using herbs, spices, marinades, sauces, and condiments. Taste-test dishes as you cook and adjust seasoning accordingly. Incorporate a variety of ingredients to add depth and complexity to flavors.

Portion Control:
Issue: Difficulty portioning meals appropriately, leading to overeating or undereating.

Solution: Use portion control tools like measuring cups, food scales, or portion-sized containers to ensure accurate serving sizes. Pre-portion meals during meal prep to avoid overeating.

Meal Storage and Organization:
Issue: Difficulty storing and organizing prepped meals in the refrigerator or freezer.
Solution: Use clear, airtight containers or meal prep containers to store meals. Label containers with the name of the dish and the date it was prepared for easy identification. Organize meals by type or mealtime to streamline meal selection.

Budget Constraints:
Issue: Feeling that healthy meal prep is too expensive.

Solution: Plan meals based on budget-friendly ingredients, buy items in bulk or on sale, and prioritize seasonal produce. Use pantry staples like beans, lentils, rice, and canned tomatoes to stretch meals further.

Motivation and Consistency:
Issue: Struggling to stay motivated and consistent with meal prep.
Solution: Set realistic goals, create a meal prep schedule, and establish a routine. Find inspiration from cooking blogs, recipe books, and social media. Involve family members or friends in meal prep to make it a shared activity.

CONCLUSION

In conclusion, the "Healthy Meal Prep Cookbook 2024" offers a comprehensive guide to mastering the art of meal prepping for optimal health and convenience. With a focus on nutritious ingredients, efficient techniques, and delicious recipes, this cookbook empowers readers to take control of their eating habits and achieve their wellness goals.

Throughout these pages, readers have discovered the benefits of meal prep, including saving time, reducing stress, and maintaining a balanced diet. They've learned essential skills such as meal planning, batch cooking, and portion control, setting them up for success in the kitchen and beyond.

From vibrant salads and hearty soups to flavorful stir-fries and satisfying snacks, the cookbook showcases a diverse array of recipes to suit every palate and dietary preference. Whether you're vegetarian, vegan, gluten-free, or following a low-carb or keto lifestyle, there's something for everyone in these pages.

As we navigate the ever-evolving landscape of health and nutrition, the "Healthy Meal Prep Cookbook 2024" serves as a trusted resource, providing timeless principles and innovative ideas to support your journey towards better eating habits and overall wellness. With practical tips, mouthwatering recipes, and a dash of inspiration, this cookbook invites readers to embrace the joy of cooking and the rewards of nourishing their bodies with wholesome, homemade meals.

Here's to a future filled with vibrant health, delicious food, and the satisfaction of knowing that you've taken proactive steps towards living your best life through the power of meal prep. Happy cooking, happy eating, and here's to your health!

We are grateful that you are starting this gastronomic adventure with the "Healthy Meal Prep Cookbook 2024." Your dedication to taking care of your body and putting your health first is incredibly motivating. Purchasing this cookbook is a proactive step towards adopting a more health-conscious lifestyle and changing your eating habits.

I hope you find plenty of tasty recipes, useful meal prep advice, and inspiration to keep you cooking as you turn through the pages of this cookbook. By working together, we're changing how we think about food and making it simpler than ever to put health first without compromising convenience or taste.

We are incredibly appreciative of your support
and happy to accompany you on your path to
healthier eating and general wellbeing. I hope
your future meals will be full of nutrition,
happiness, and the fulfillment that comes from
knowing that you're caring for your body from
the inside out. Here's to many happy and
healthy meals.

We appreciate that you have selected the
"Healthy Meal Prep Cookbook 2024." To your
well-being and prosperity, cheers!